# Passion flower & Fruit: Toxic Riddles for Toxic Detective

# AN INDIAN SOCIETY OF TOXICOLOGY INITIATIVE

For Crime Scene Investigators (CSi), Toxicologists, Police Officers, CID, CBI officers, Lawyers, Judges, Magistrates, Legal counsels, Students, Forensic Scientists, Doctors, Toxicology Nurses & Emergency Paramedics

Dr Vivekanshu Verma, MBBS, Postgraduate Diploma in Forensic Medicine & Toxicology, Fellow of Indian Society of Toxicology, Associate consultant, Emergency & Trauma care, Medanta-The Medicity, Gurugram. Honorary Toxicology Expert, Central Bureau of Investigation

Dr Vijay Vasudev Pillay, MBBS, MD Forensic Medicine & Toxicology, Chief, Poison Control Centre, Professor & Head, Forensic Medicine & Toxicology, Amrita School of Medicine, Amrita Vishwa Vidyapeetham, Cochin, Kerala

Dr Shiv Rattan Kochar, MBBS, MD Forensic Medicine & Toxicology, Senior Professor, Forensic Medicine. Chief Vigilance Officer, Metro MANAS Arogya Sadan Heart Care & Multispecialty Hospital, Directorate of Medical Education, Jaipur (Rajasthan)

Dr Prateek Rastogi, MBBS. MD, HOD & Professor, Department of Forensic Medicine & Toxicology, Kasturba Medical College, Mangalore, Karnataka

Dr. Shweta H Patel, MBBS, MD Forensic Medicine & Toxicology, Assistant Professor, Forensic Medicine & Toxicology, Pramukhswami Medical College, Karamsad. Dist. Anand, Gujarat.

# PASSION FLOWER & FRUIT: TOXIC RIDDLES FOR TOXIC DETECTIVE: AN INDIAN SOCIETY OF TOXICOLOGY INITIATIVE

1st Edition, 2020

ISBN: 9798564444460

©2020 Indian Society of Toxicology

# PUBLISHED BY POISON CONTROL CENTRE

Amrita Institute of Medical Science,

Ponekkara, P. O, Kochi, Kerala - 682041.

# PASSIONFLOWER: PASSIFLORA

192nd Toxic Riddle in rhymes
Get Harm in, Pass I, on wine
Toxicity may pop, to live, are
Benzo flaw won harm all dine
Malt all, drank in tea for bar
Night, insomnia starts to set
The ache builds in tummy for
U know that U must go to bed
And you try to take some rest
hug tears stained pillow close
When no one is anyway around
And cries for one u loved & lost
And screams without a sound
Others see you in a bright day
And thinks you are doing well
But every day as evening sets
I see you enter your own hell
Time hasn't healed u at all
Or quieted your own fears

So every night, alone in bed

You shed your silent tears

Consuming me, as you said

# PASSION CRUCIFIED

Passionflower is a beautiful, exotic looking plant that's known for its soothing effects on body and mind.

The medicinal benefits of passion flower weren't widely recognized until the 19th century, but it's been used by native people groups of North and South America for centuries.

The common name "passion flower" comes from Spanish missionaries who thought that it resembled a crucifix.

It was known by the Spanish as 'La Flor de las Cinco Llagas' or the 'The Flower With The Five Wounds.' 'Passionis' refers to Christ's passion, representing various elements of the Crucifixion.

It became symbolic of the whole crucifixion story of Jesus Christ, which is also referred to as "the Passion."

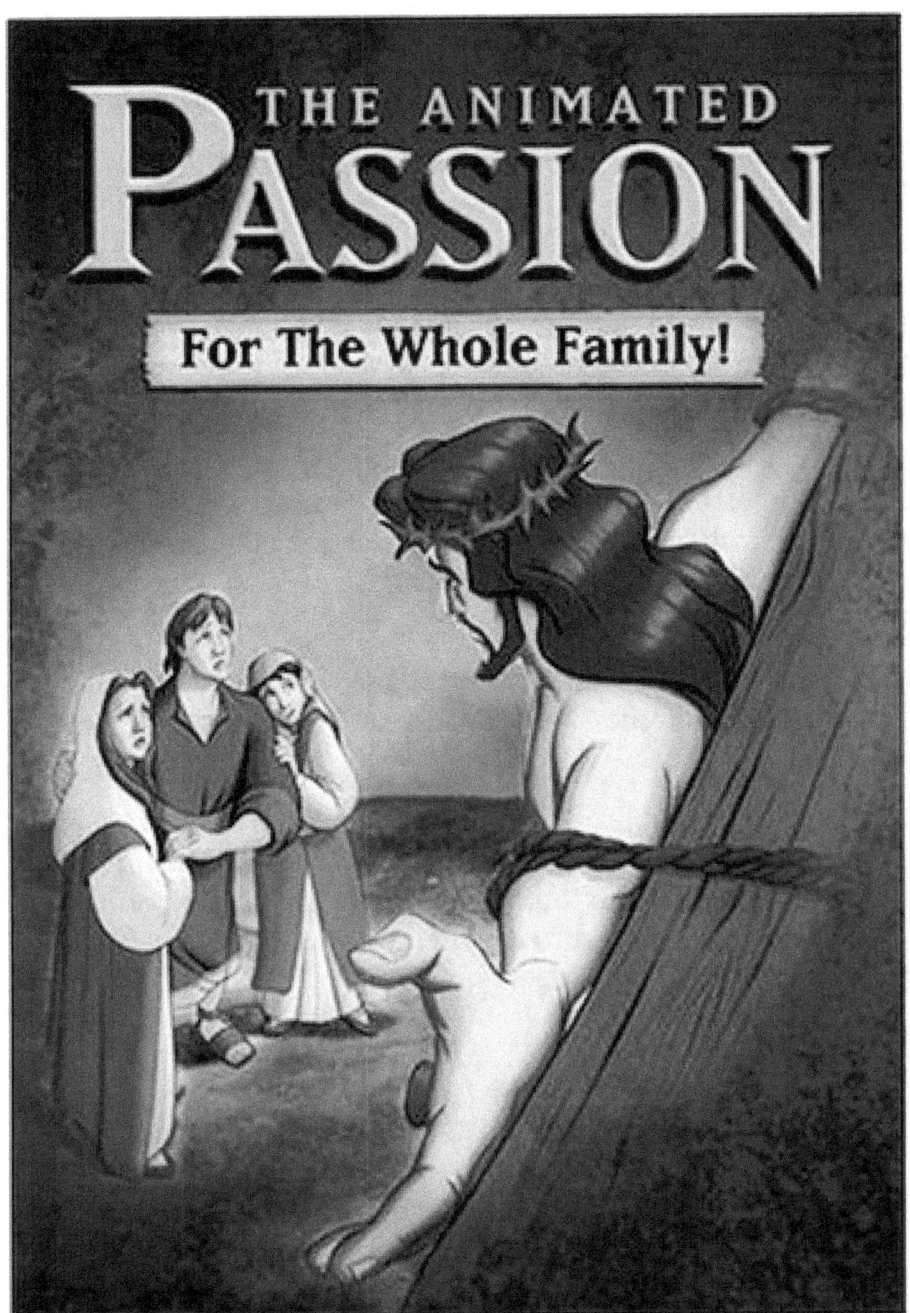

Figure 1. The Animated Passion: Biblical story(2004). Passion (Actor), Richard Rich (Director)

# MYTHOLOGY

The passion flower is associated with Christ, because several parts of this flower represent different aspects of the crucifixion.

For example, the spiraled tendrils in the center of the flower symbolize the lash marks Christ received while being whipped prior to the crucifixion.

The central flower column is a symbol of the whip that was used to lash Christ, and the 72 radial filaments represent the crown of thorns.

Also, the top three stigmas of the flower symbolize the three nails used during the crucifixion, and the lower five anthers symbolize the five wounds that resulted from the nails.

# PASSION OF CHRIST

THE PASSION OF THE CHRIST focuses on the last 12 hours of Jesus of Nazareth's life.

The mythological story primarily covers the final 12 hours before Jesus' death, consisting of the Passion, hence the title of the film.

It begins with the Agony in the Garden in the Garden of Olives (or Gethsemane), the betrayal of Judas Iscariot, the brutal Scourging at the Pillar, the suffering of Mary as prophesied by Simeon, the crucifixion and death of Christ, and ends with a brief depiction of his resurrection.

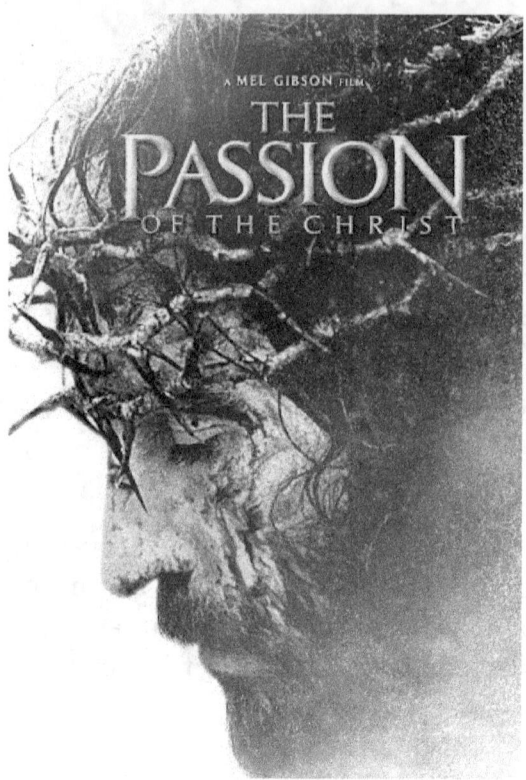

Figure 2. The Passion of the Christ is 2004 American biblical drama film produced, co-written and directed by Mel Gibson

A principal source is The Dolorous Passion of Our Lord Jesus Christ, the visions of Anne Catherine Emmerich (1774–1824), as written by the poet Clemens Brentano.

Ref: Jesus and Mel Gibson's The Passion of the Christ by Kathleen E. Corley, Robert Leslie Webb. 2004

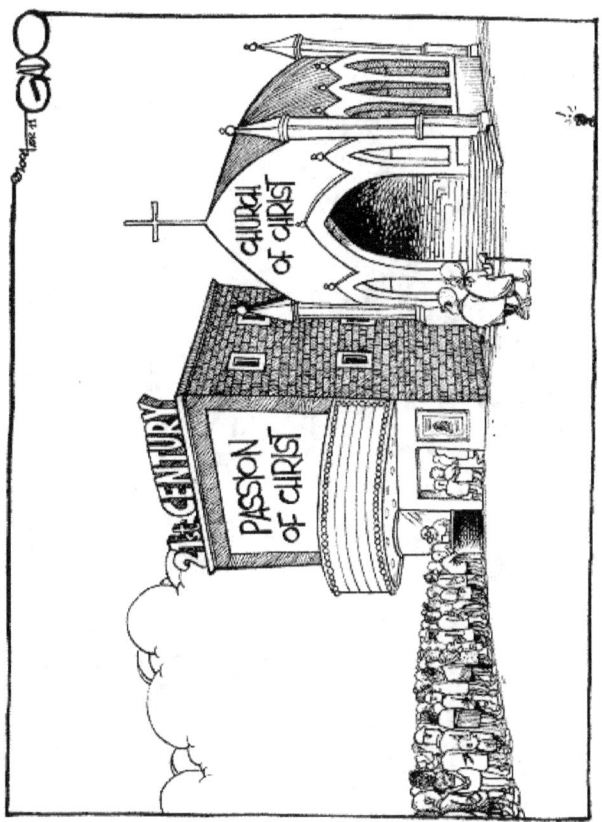

Figure 3. Passion of Christ.

The following cartoon appeared in the Easter Sunday edition of the Daily Nation, the major newspaper in Kenya, East Africa, soon after "The Passion of Christ" appeared in theatres. The drawing contrasted the "Passion" and "Church" of Christ (Sunday Nation, April 11).

Link: http://www.missiology.org/blog/GVR-MR-33-Imagining-Christs-Church-in-the-City

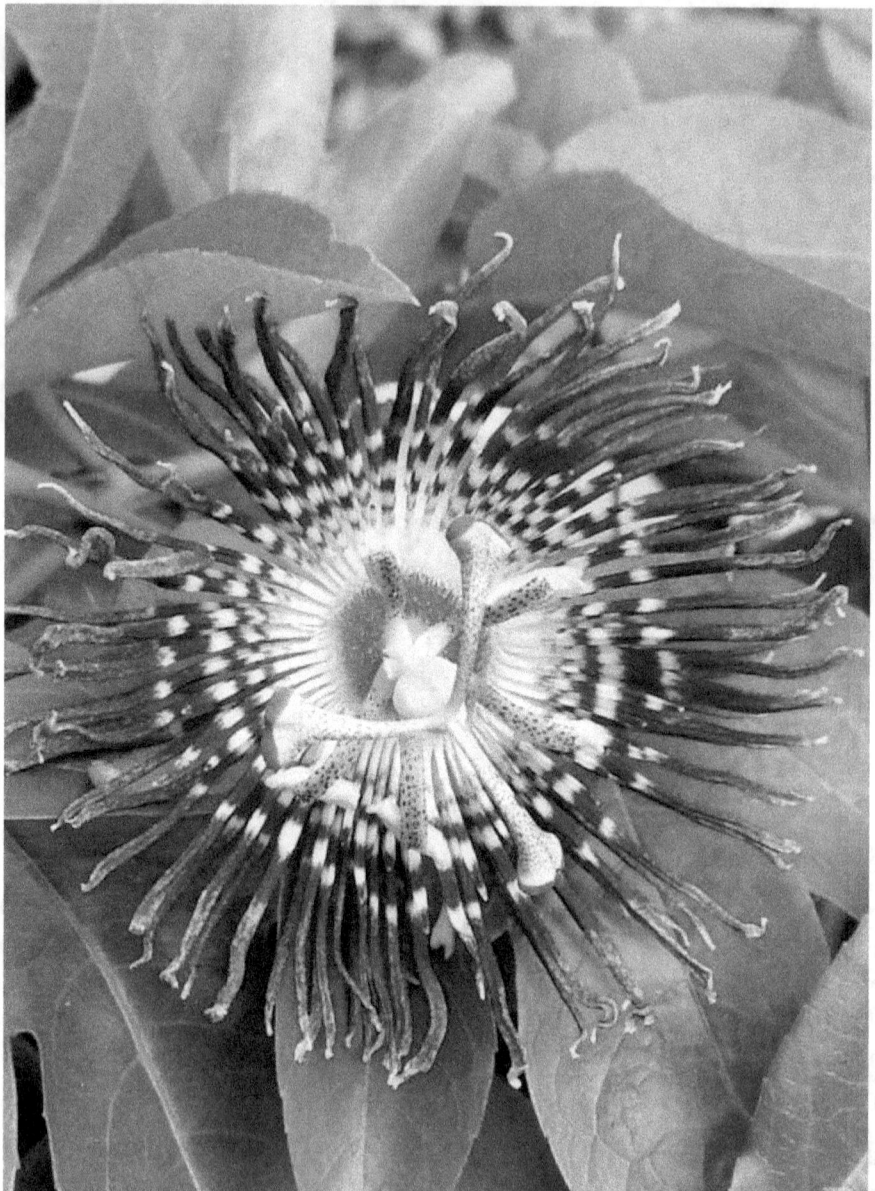

Figure 4. Passion flower:

# PASSION FLOWER & FRUIT: TOXIC RIDDLES FOR TOXIC DETECTIVE

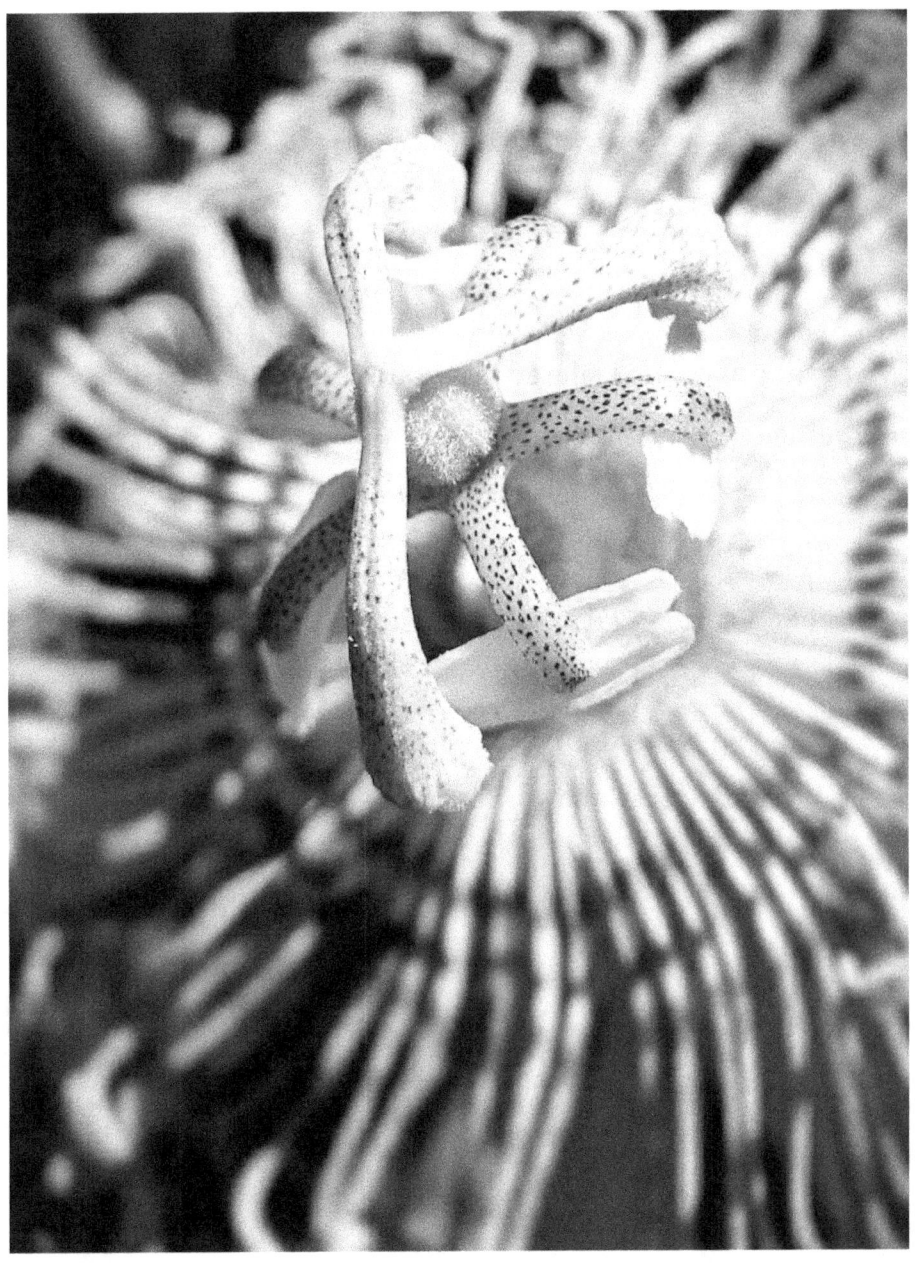

# KRISHAN-KAMALA:

**Krishna: Indian Lord of Passion**
Why Passionflower is related mythological to Lord Krishna?

It is believed with reference of Hindu epic 'Mahabharata' that:

- There are about 100 of blue petals – one for each of the Kauravas.

- 5 of the yellow ones in the centre – one for each of the Pandavas.

- The green bulb in the centre symbolises Draupadi, the queen of Pandava,

- The three filaments are for the holy trinity of Brahma-Vishnu-Shiva and,

- The radial in the centre is the Sudarshan Chakra of Lord Krishna.

- Its colour, fragrance, shape, the vine, the leaves; everything about it is simply unique and magically beautiful.

## PASSION FLOWER & FRUIT: TOXIC RIDDLES FOR TOXIC DETECTIVE

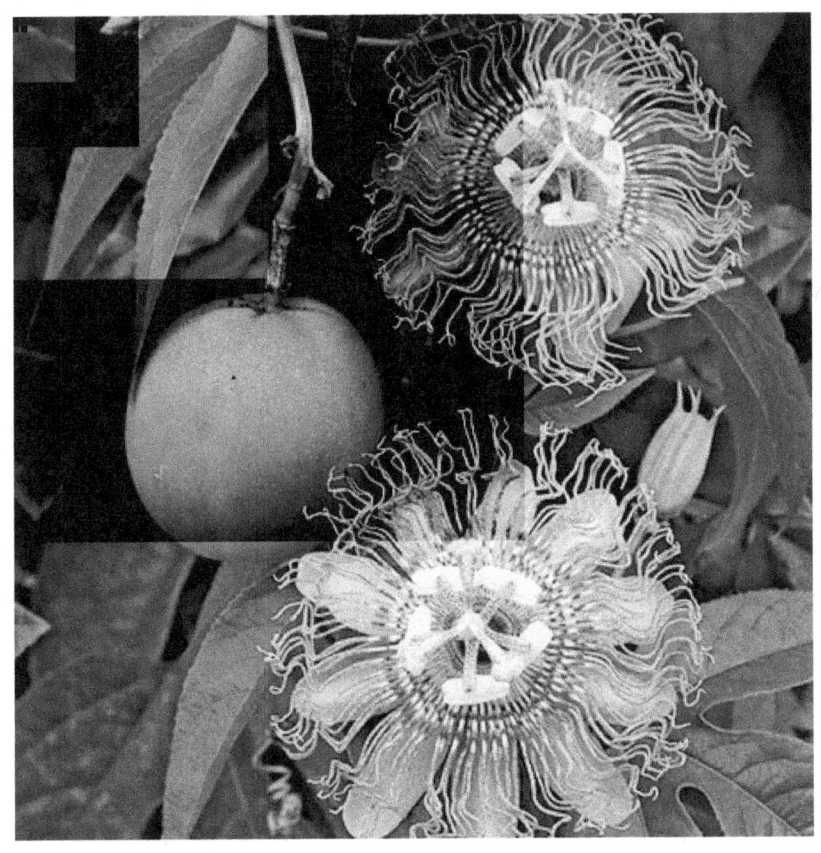

# PANCH PANDAV

In India, blue passionflowers are called Krishna kamala (कृष्णकमळ) in Karnataka and Maharashtra, while in Uttar Pradesh and generally north it is colloquially called "Panch Pandav" (referring to the five Pandavas in the Hindu epic, the Mahabharata).

The five anthers are interpreted as the five Pandavas, the divine Krishna is at the centre, and the radial filaments are opposing hundred.

The colour blue is moreover associated with Krishna as the colour of his aura.

# RAKHI: CHAKRA OF SUDARSHAN

On an auspicious day, Lord Ganesha's sister Manasa visits him to tie him a rakhi.

Rakshabandhan or Rakhi, is a popular festival in India which is celebrated on the day of Shravan Poornima.

This day, sister tie sacred threads on the wrists of their brothers wishing good health and long life to them.

Following incident is mentioned in the Mahabharata.

According to one version on a Sankranti day, Krishna to cut his little finger while handling sugarcane. Sathyabama, his queen immediately sent her help to get a bandage cloth while his other consort, Rukmini rushed to bring some cloth herself.

Draupadi who was nearby, tore off a part of her sari and bandaged his finger. In return for this deed, Krishna promised to protect her in time of distress.

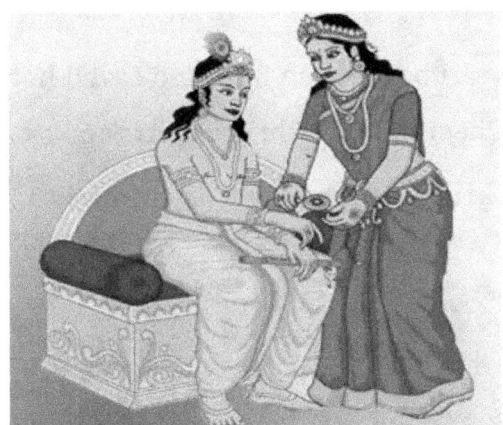

Figure 5. Rakshabandhan – Krishna and Draupadi story

There is an another narrative related to this incident which says that while killing Shisupala, Krishna, held the lightning fast Sudarshana on his finger and sent it the king's way. Within a second, Shishupala was beheaded.

Lord Krishna's finger started bleeding and Draupadi, an ardent devotee of the Lord and the Pandavas' wife, rushed to bandage the bleeding finger of her beloved Lord. She tore a small piece from her sari and tied it to the Lord's hand.

Krishna was touched by this selfless token of affection and pledged to rush to Draupadi's protection whenever needed. Draupadi used to tie a rakhi to the Lord's hand every year and Krishna always showered His protection on her.

The word he is said to have uttered is 'Akshyam' which was a boon meaning 'unending'.

And that was how Draupadi's sari became endless and saved her embarrassment on the day of Cheerharan in Dhritarashtra's court.
Link: http://ritsin.com/rakhi-krishna-draupadi-story.html/

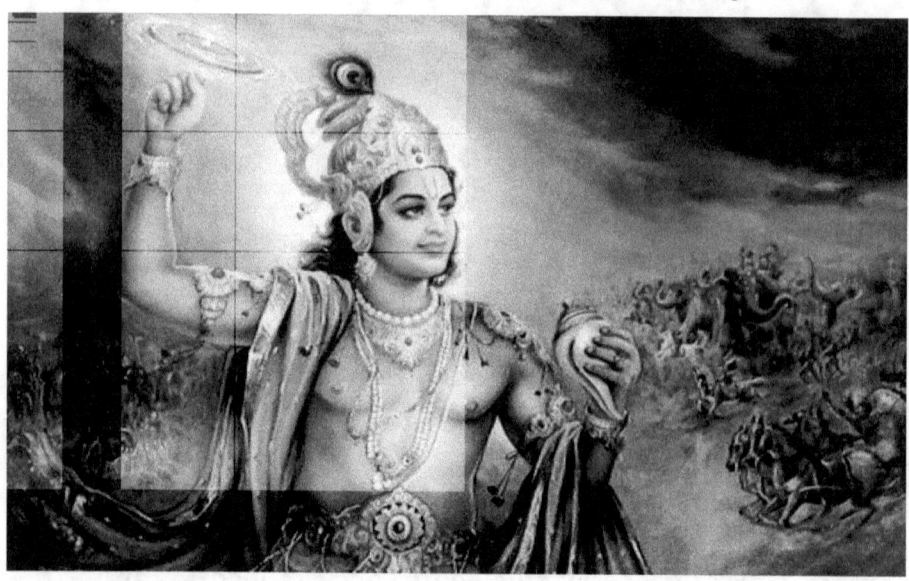

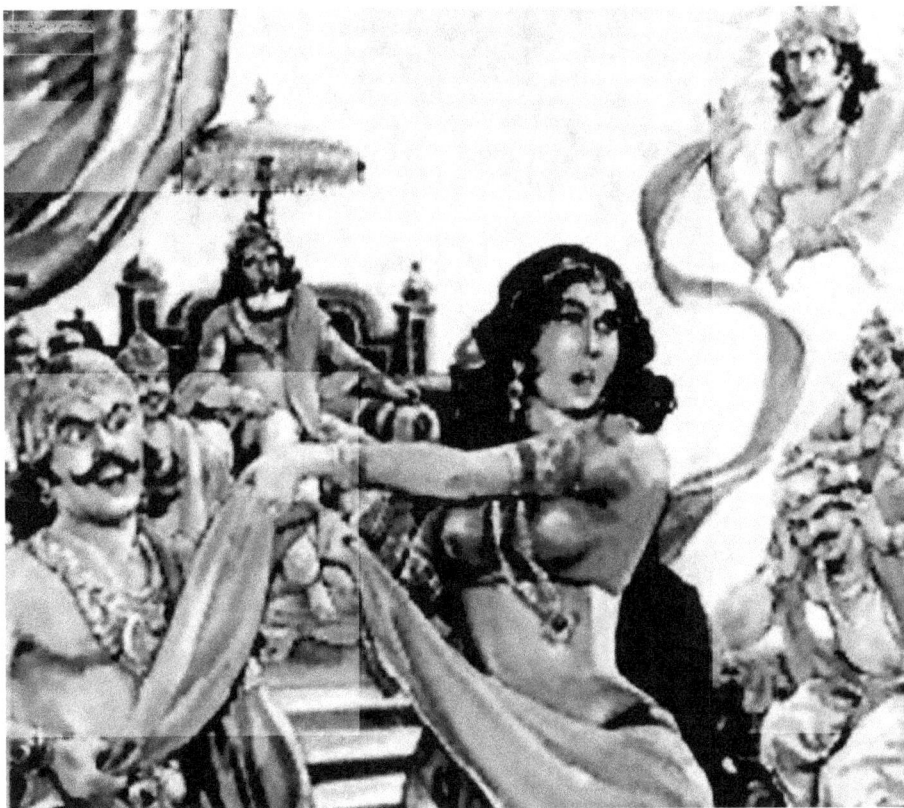

Figure 6. **Mahabharata Draupadi Vastraharan (Disrobing) and Lord Krishna Saving her, A unforatabble momement of Mahabharata**

Arjuna being a bother-in-law of Lord Krishna by his marriage to Lord Krishna's foster sister Subhadre, Krishne (Draupadi) also becomes a sister for Lord Krishna.

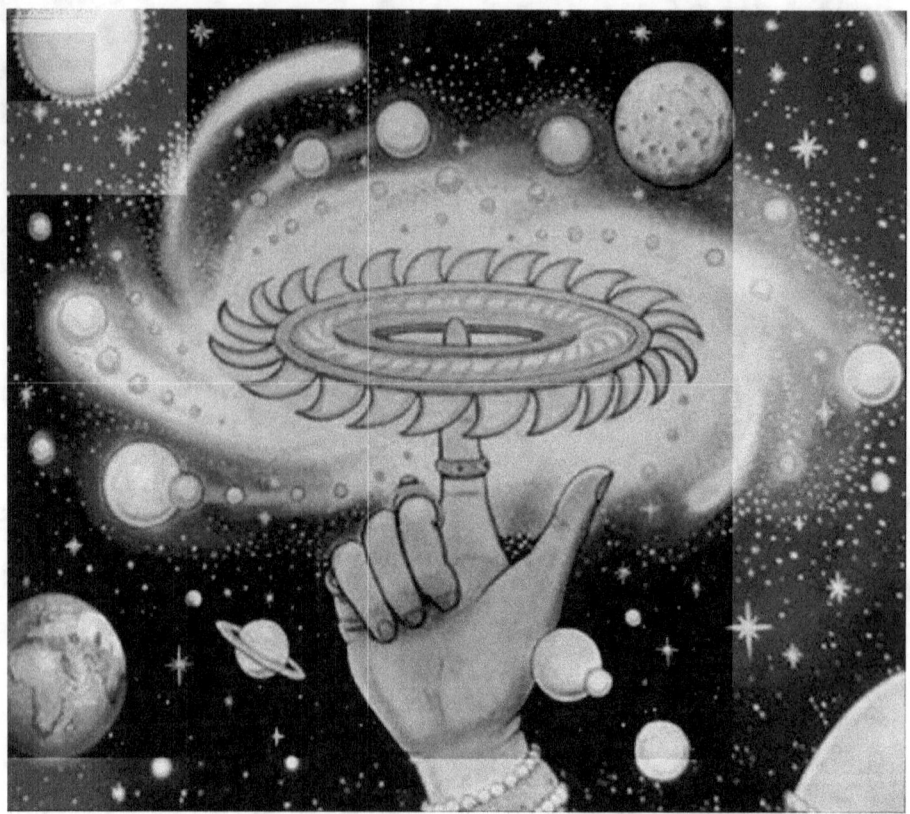

Figure 7. Sudarshan Chakra

Nobel laureate Rabindranath Tagore started a mass Raksha Bandhan festival during the Partition of Bengal (1905), in which he encouraged Hindu and Muslim women to tie a rakhi on men from the other community and make them their brothers.

Link: https://www.hindustantimes.com/more-lifestyle/raksha-bandhan-2019-significance-facts-and-history-of-the-festival/story-CgDtNFp8ZBwpPb6TuxzRrO.html

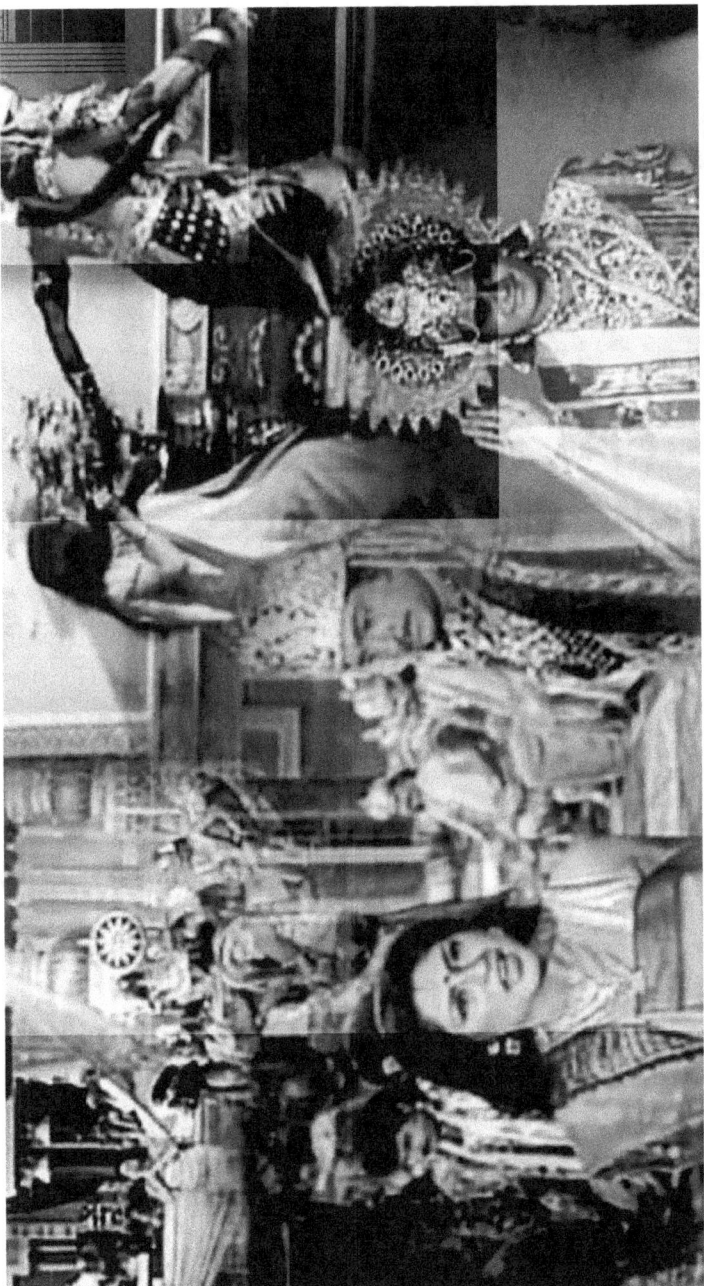

Figure 8. Mahabharata serial by Director BR Chopra depicted the mythological significance

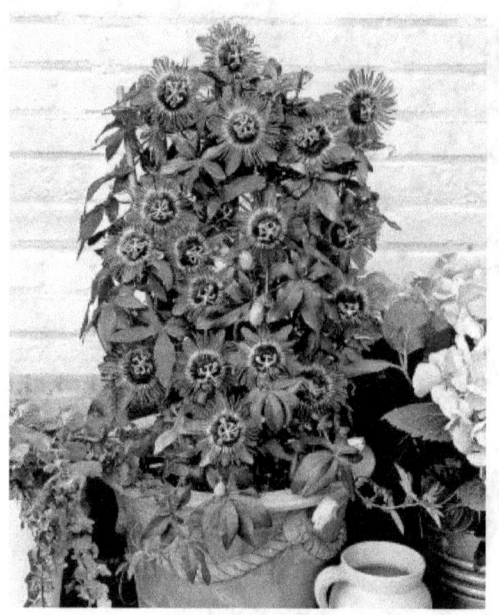

Source: Krishna Kamal – Why is Passion Flower Named After The God? By The Solo Globetrotter (2016). https://blog.nurserylive.com/2016/08/25/krishna-kamal-why-is-passion-flower-named-after-the-god-and-gardening-in-india

**Kaurav Pandav Flower**

This flower also resembles a Rakhi: holy sacred wrist band which is worn on the wrist of every brother on Raksha Bandhan festival all over India as the symbol of a sister's love for her brother, first tied by Draupadi to Lord Krishna, who saved her dignity later during Mahabharata's infamous dice game losing & disrobing act of Dushasana.

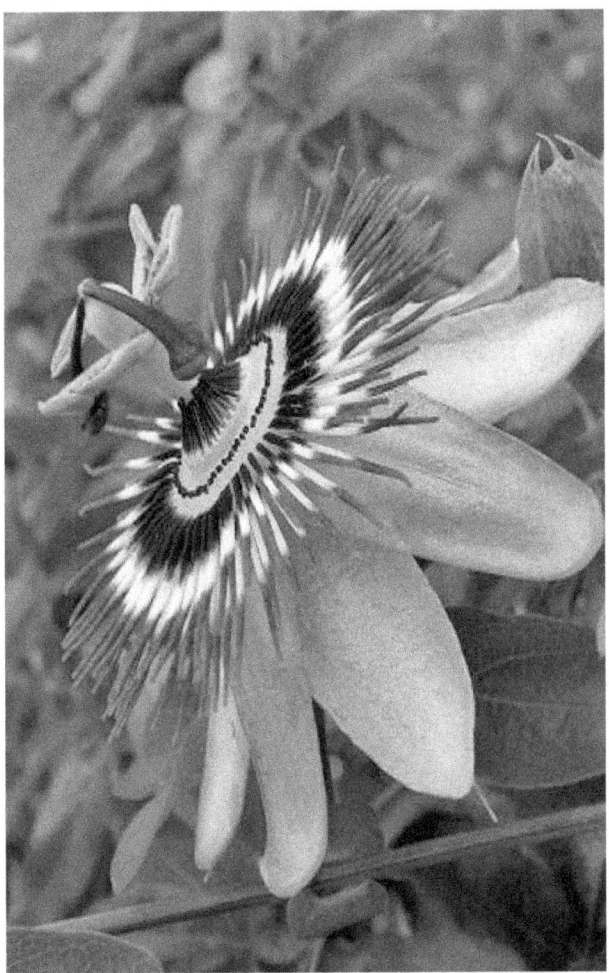

**Common name:** Soi Fah Passion Flower

- **Hindi**: झुमका लता Jhumkalata

Link: https://www.patrika.com/jabalpur-news/amazing-facts-about-kaurav-pandav-flower-read-here-1303883/

# HISTORY

The plant family Passifloraceae was defined by Jussieu in 1805 and is currently subdivided into 650 species and 16 genera.

Predominantly occurring in America and tropical Africa, it was probably discovered by Monardes, a Spanish doctor who described the plant in Peru in 1569.

# RIDDLE ANALYSIS

**Answer:**

Passiflora known in Hindi as ( कृष्ण कमल ) Krishan-Kamala, (also known in English as maypop, apricot vine, passion vine, and purple passion flower) is most often referred to as "passion flower" and seems, in recent research at least, to be considered the most medicinally active member of the Passifloraceae family.

Since the sixteenth century, if a patient was tossing and turning at night, worried, or had a nervous stomach, and was getting no sleep, there was a simple remedy that physicians were very likely to prescribe: a tea or tincture of passionflower.

Herbalists and some doctors will still recommend it but, from a scientific standpoint, the remedy does not seem so simple as it once did.

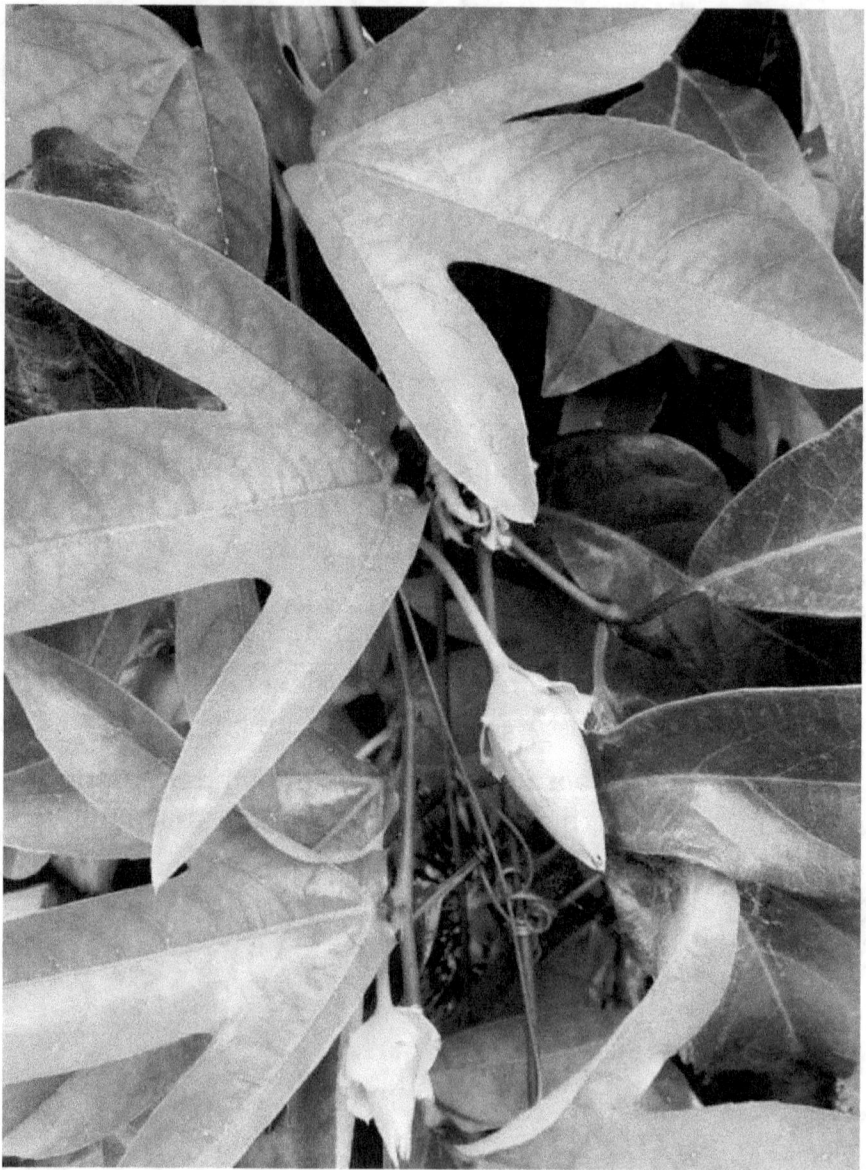

Figure 9. Buds & leaves of Passiflora. Image Source: TPS Kumar

Passionflower is a name that has been given to several members of the genus Passiflora.

There are more than 40 species in the genus whose origins are in both the tropical and subtropical regions of the western hemisphere.

A species of Passiflora was first brought to Europe from Mexico in the sixteenth century by Spanish conquerors.

Not long after this plant's importation, it gained favor as a calming herbal tea. It is now part of the medicinal herbarium in many countries throughout the world.

This herb was named passionflower because various parts of the plant were seen as symbols of Christ' s scourging, crowning with thorns, and crucifixion.

Passionflower's long history in herbal medicine includes its use as a treatment for colic, diarrhea, dysentery, menstrual pain, skin eruptions, conjunctivitis, hemorrhoids, and muscle spasms

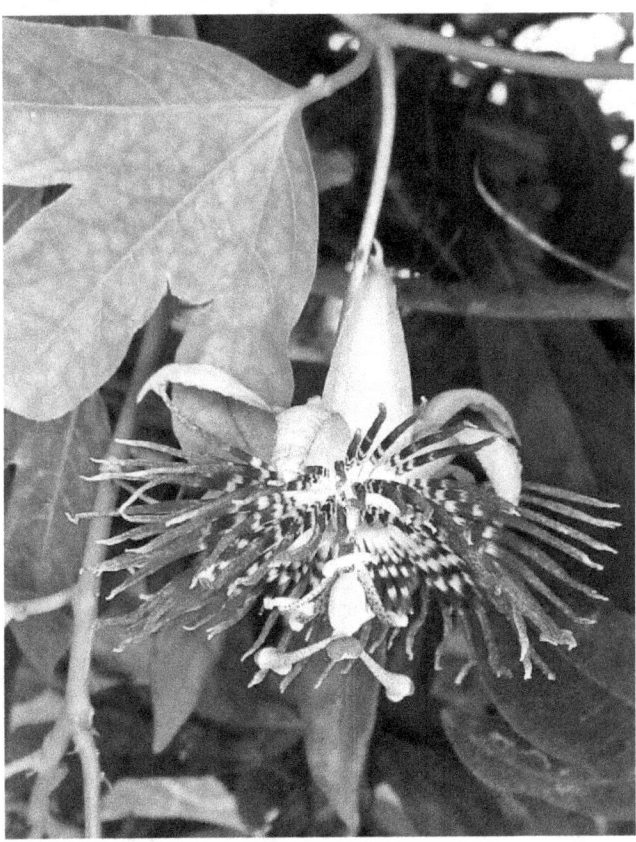

Figure 10. Flower of Passiflora. Image Source: TPS Kumar

# TAXONOMIC CONFUSION

One of the problems with this subtropical plant is its identity.

Passionflower is a name that has been applied to a number of species in the Passiflora genus.

There is a lot of confusion about several of the species' names.

Passiflora edulis, has often been confused with P. incarnata and the names, have been used synonymously.

The word passiflora is from the Latin and means "passion flower."

In Brazil, these plant family is known as "maracuja," a word from the Tupi-Guarani' language.


Cronin JR. 2003. Passionflower Reigniting male libido and other potential uses. Altern Complement Ther 9 89–92.

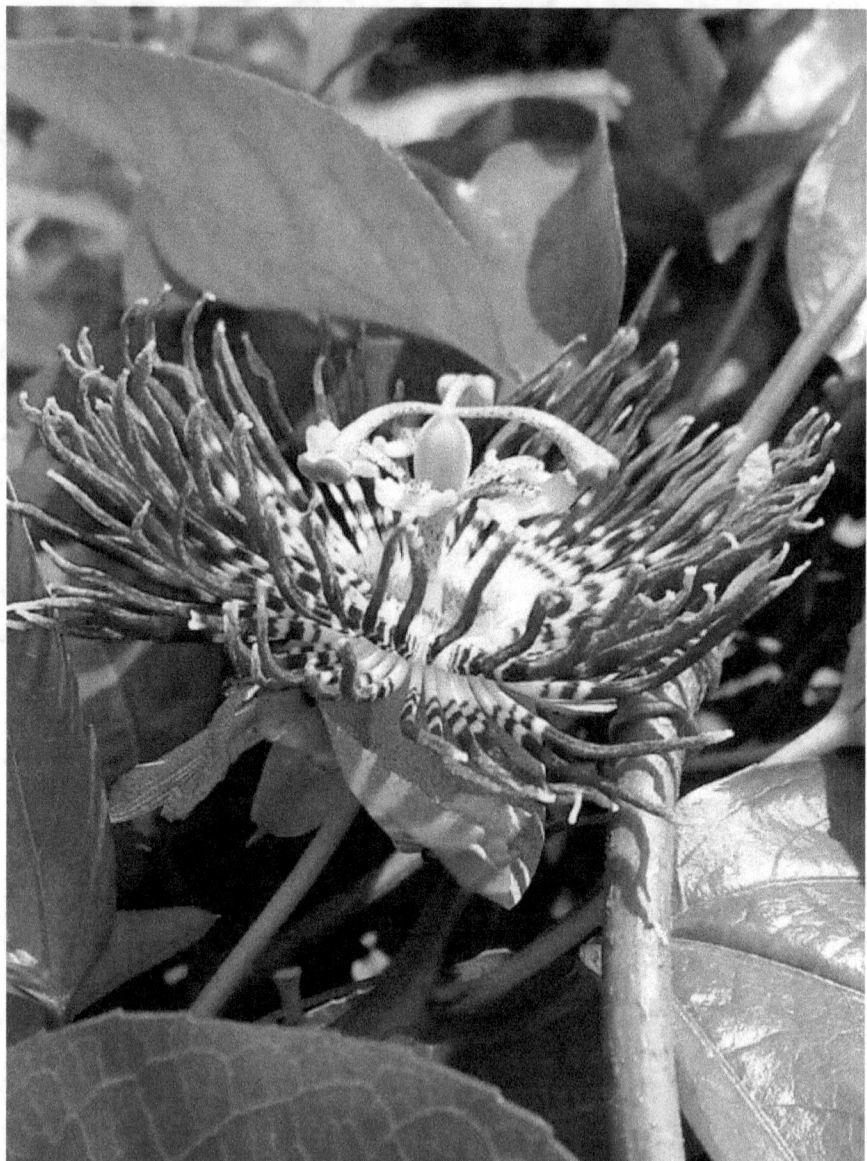

Figure 11. Purple Flower

Its major use is an edible fruit, but its extracts are used in various medications.

# BOTANY

Passion flower, is a dynamic climbing plant which utilizes tendrils in its upward growth.

It has woody stems reaching up to 8-9 meters.

It blooms with large and striking flowers that are typically blue-purple.

They are mostly tendril-bearing vines, with some being shrubs or trees. They can be woody or herbaceous. Passion flowers produce regular and usually showy flowers with a distinctive corona.

The flower is pentamerous and ripens into an indehiscent fruit with numerous seeds.

An egg-shaped fruit will develop that ripens from green to yellow and is eaten by both humans and wildlife.

Passiflora incarnata is an evergreen climber, rapidly growing up to 6 m (19 ft 8 in).

This plant is in leaf from December to January, in flower from June to July, and its seeds ripen from September to November.

This plant possesses hermaphrodite flowers (possessing both male and female organs) which are pollinated by insects such as bees.

Passiflora incarnata can grow in light (sandy), medium (loamy) or heavy (clay) soils, with a preference for well-drained soil, and it cannot grow in the shade due to the soil moisture in shady areas.

Description of the different parts of the plant:

- Stems – Vining, glabrous to minutely pubescent,

herbaceous. Tendrils present.
- Leaves – Alternate, 3-lobed, serrulate, petiolate, up to 15 cm long, 13 cm wide, glabrous. Petioles with two glands near the base of the leaf blade.
- Inflorescence – Single pedicillate flowers from leaf axils.
- Flowers – A corona consisting of a structure of appendages situated between the corolla and the stamens. As shown in the graphical abstract, the corona is the ring-like structure of purple and white appendages above the petals and sepals. The flower is typically 6–7 cm in diameter. The flower has 5 petals and 5 sepals, which are purplish to whitish, similar, and alternating. The flower has 3 styles, typically 3 stamens, 5 greenish-white sepals with terminal appendages.
- Fruit – Fleshy, ovoid to globose, initially green, yellowish-red at maturity.
- Flowering – June – September.
- Habitat – Thickets, waste ground, disturbed sites, roadsides, railroads.

# HERBAL USES

All parts (flowers, leaves, and stems) of the Passion flower are used for medicinal purposes.

In Brazil, only the use of the leaves of Passiflora alata of the variety dryander is permitted for the preparation of medications.

In a Brazilian dictionary of pharmaceutical specialties there are 20 medications containing passion flower.

It is known, however, that extracts are made also with other parts of the plant, such as the stalk, and with other varieties.

The major pharmacologic property of passiflora is depression of the central nervous system, causing sedation.

This effect was described by Phares in 1867, who used this substance for patients with insomnia and irritability.

Freitas et al(1985), who reviewed the literature, has reported other effects: hypotension, contraction of intestinal smooth muscle, bradycardia, hypothermia, skeletal muscle relaxation, and antispasmodic and anti-inflammatory effects by passiflora.

Citation: Freitas PCD. Estudo Farmagnó́stico Comparativo de Espécies Brasileiras do Genero Passiflora L. São Paulo, 1985. Tese de mestrado da Faculdade de Ciências Farmaceuticas da Universidade de São Paulo—n. 615.323.456.

# NEELKAMAL

## *Beautiful Catch of Rakhiflower*

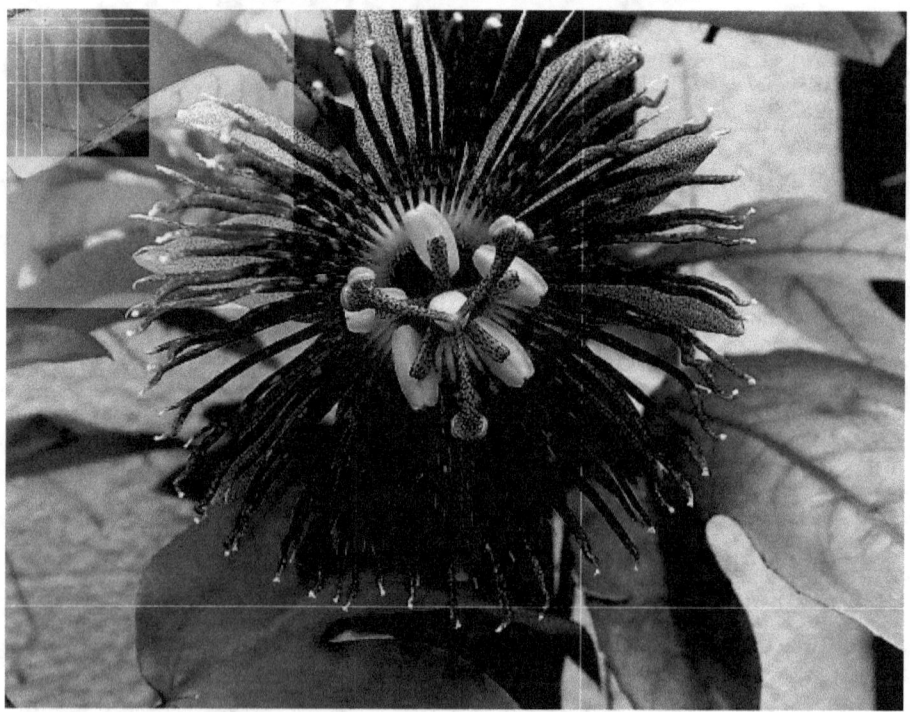

Figure 12. Neelkamal or KrishnaKamal: Rakhiflower

## PASSION FLOWER & FRUIT: TOXIC RIDDLES FOR TOXIC DETECTIVE

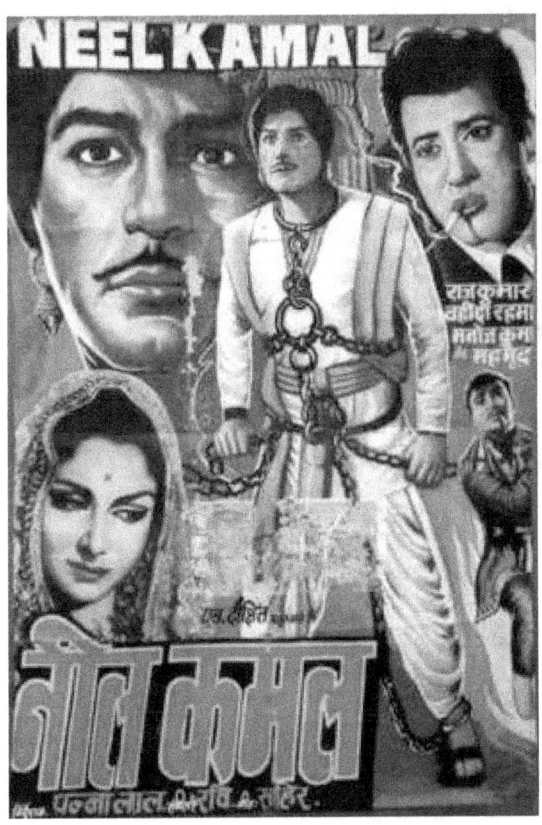

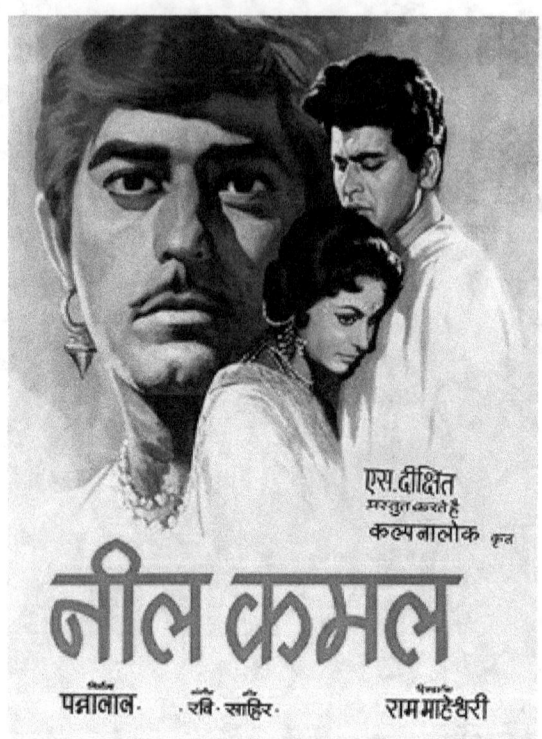

This is a poster for Neel Kamal (1968 film).

# SUGGESTIONS AND CAVEATS

Practitioners have traditionally prescribed passionflower to treat minor problems with anxiety or muscle spasms.

For these purposes, there seem to be no additional warnings. With regard to more recent treatment suggestions (e.g., as a male libido enhancer or as an adjuvant for treating drug withdrawal symptoms), perhaps some restraint in expectations would be appropriate, given the small amount of data available.

With regard to the prospect of uncovering passionflower's "active principle," particularly for treating CNS-related effects, there may be some developments soon, especially in light of the fact that the flowers and root appear to be devoid of activity.

This is one case in which scientific inquiry seems to offer the possibility of refining a traditional plant extract.

Yet, the old principle of using the plant material or simple extracts is likely to produce beneficial synergistic effects that isolation of single constituents may not provide.

Cronin JR. 2003. Passionflower Reigniting male libido and other potential uses. Altern Complement Ther 9 89–92.

Main flavonoids as secondary compounds of *Passiflora incarnata* L. phytocomplex.

| Flavonoid | Molecular formula | Skeletal formula |
|---|---|---|
| Chrysin | $C_{15}H_{10}O_4$ | |
| Vitexin | $C_{21}H_{20}O_{10}$ | |
| Isovitexin | $C_{21}H_{20}O_{10}$ | |
| Orientin | $C_{21}H_{20}O_{11}$ | |
| Isoorientin | $C_{21}H_{20}O_{11}$ | |
| Apigenin | $C_{15}H_{10}O_5$ | |
| Kaempferol | $C_{15}H_{10}O_6$ | |

Figure 13. Structure of flavonoids in Passiflora incarnate. Image Source: M. Miroddi et al. / Journal of Ethnopharmacology 150 (2013) 791–804.

# BENZOFLAVONE

BENZO FLAW WON HARM ALL DINE

Benzo fla vone = Benzoflavone (homophonic)

Harmol = harm all (homophonic)

Some researchers have ascribed the sedative effects of P. incarnata to indole alkaloids such as harmane and its relatives harmaline and harmol.

Citation: Lutomski, J., 1960. Isolation der Wichtigsten Alkaloide aus dem Kranz der Passionsblume (P. incarnata). Biuletyn Instytut Roslin Leczniczych 6, 209–219.

Other researchers have suggested that P. incarnata's alkaloid content is too small to cause this and other CNS effects and that flavonoids— such as apigenin, luteolin, or scopoletin or their glycosides—are more likely to account for CNS bioactivity.

Citation: Speroni E, Minghetti A. Neuropharmacological activity of extracts from Passiflora incarnata. Planta Med 1988;54:488–491.

Still other researchers report results that support neither of these phytochemical types in the neuropharmacologic activity of P. incarnata extract.

Citation: Soulimani R, et al. Behavioral effects of Passiflora incarnata L. and its indole alkaloid and flavonoid derivatives and maltol in the mouse. J Ethnopharmacol 1997;57:11–20.


A recent paper described the isolation of an apparently highly anxiolytic, trisubstituted benzoflavone moiety from a P. incarnata extract.

Citation: Dhawan K, et al. Anti-anxiety studies on extracts of Passiflora incarnata Linneaus. J Ethnopharmacol 2001;78:165–170.


Unfortunately, the identity of this benzoflavone will be under wraps while the research group involved with the study pursues patent rights.

# VITEXIN & ISOVITEXIN

Vitexin is an apigenin flavone glycoside, which is found in the passion flower, Vitex agnus-castus (chaste tree or chasteberry), in the Phyllostachys nigra bamboo leaves, in the pearl millet (Pennisetum millet), and in Hawthorn.

Vitexin has a role as a platelet aggregation inhibitor, an alpha-glucosidase inhibitor, an antineoplastic agent and a plant metabolite.

Isovitexin (or homovitexin, saponaretin) is a flavone.

Isovitexin can be found in the passion flower, Cannabis, and the açaí palm.

Lutomski, J., Adamska, M., 1968. Isolation of vitexin from the flavonoid fraction of Passiflora incarnata L. Herba Polonia 14, 249.

Isovitexin

Vitexin

Figure 14. Vitexin & Isovitexin structure. Source: https://pubchem.ncbi.nlm.nih.gov/compound/Vitexin

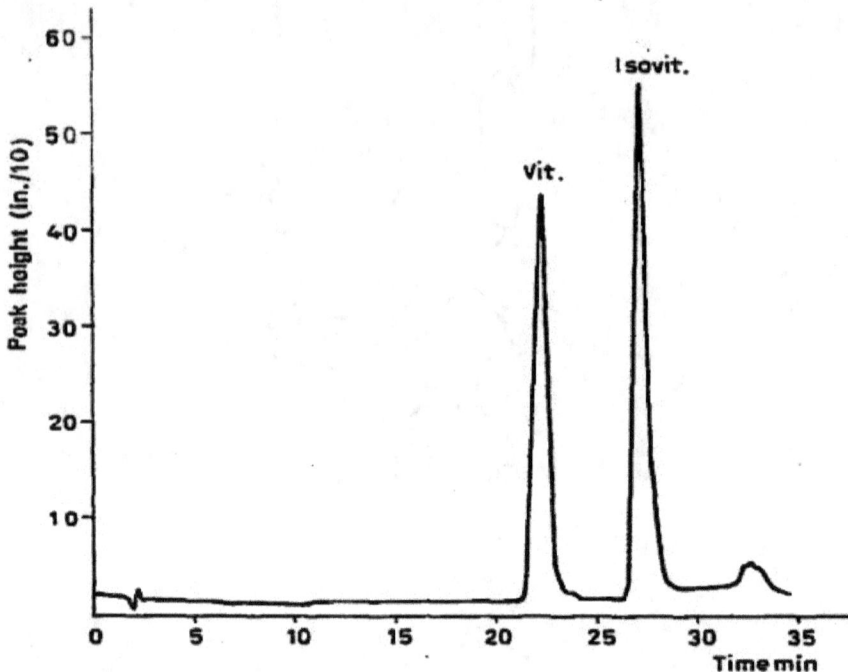

Figure 15. Separation of vitexin and isovitexin standards on a Zorbax ODS column. Source: J. Chromatog. 161, 396–402.

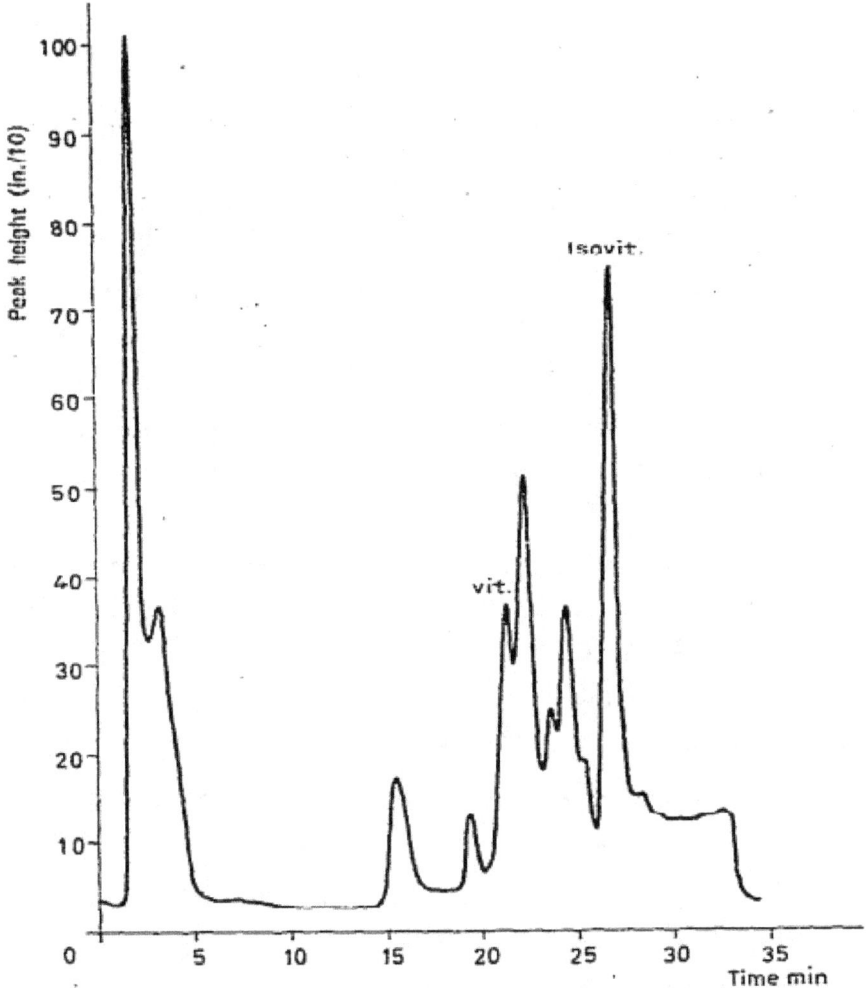

Figure 16. Chrornatogram of a methznolic solution of Passiflora incamata pilular extract. Source: J. Chromatog. 161, 396–402.

Quercia, V., 1978. Identification and determination of vitexin and isovitexin in Passiflora incarnata extracts. J. Chromatog. 161, 396–402.

# HEART IN PASSION

The most intensive study of passiflora on the cardiovascular system was made by George HR et al (1940) at Laboratory of Pharmacology, College of Medicine, The Ohio State University.

These findings are of particular interest in view of the fact that the use of Passiflora in modern therapeutics is based solely on its supposed sedative action.

The carotid blood pressure was recorded to observe the effect of the active substance alone and in conjunction with other drugs having known effects.

The cardioactive substance of passiflora is inactive by mouth, and when injected intravenously its action is fleeting.

It was assumed for these reasons that the active principle was rapidly destroyed, possibly in the liver.

Doses of 1-3 mg. per Kg. body weight were injected into the femoral vein of dogs anesthetized with ether.

Immediately following the injection the blood pressure fell 40-60 mm. and rose slowly to normal.

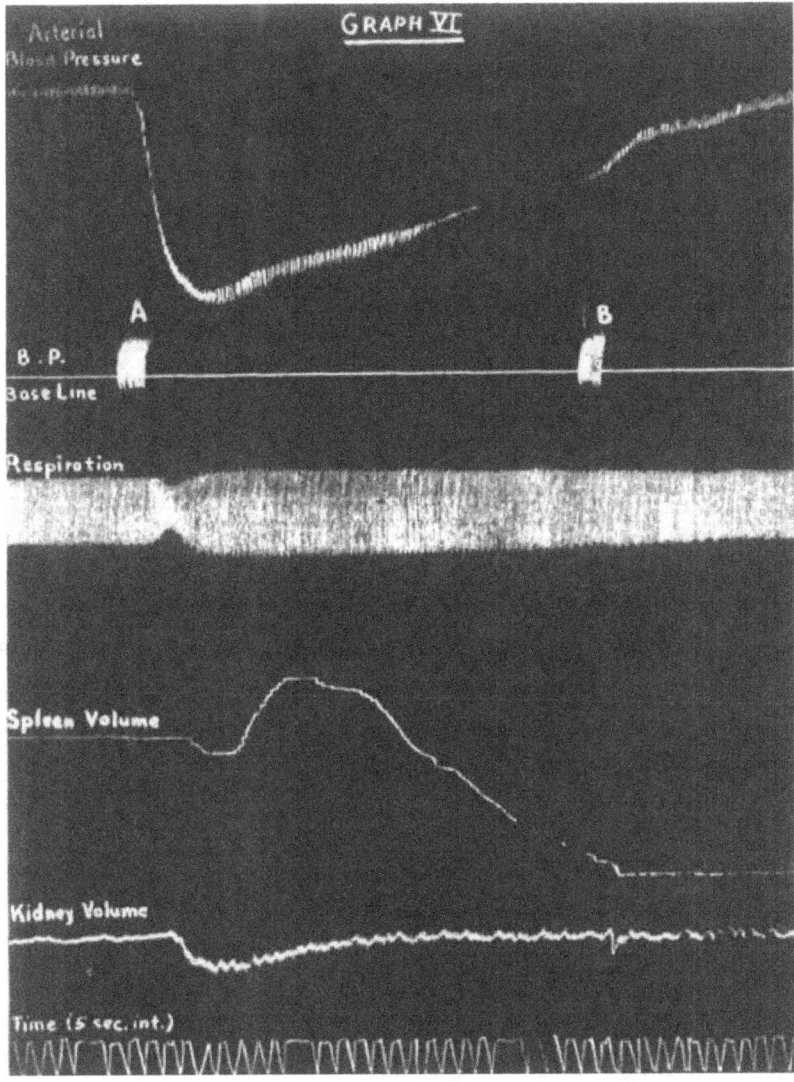

Figure 17. Changes in the Blood Pressure, Respiration, Spleen Volume and Kidney Volume Following the Injection of Passiflora extract. Source: Journal Of The American Pharmaceutical Association. Volume 29, Issue 6, 1940, Pages 245-249.

The effect of the active principle in producing a fall in blood pressure, dilatation of the heart and constriction of the smooth muscle of the intestine would seem to indicate that the active principle was parasympathotropic.

However, this is not universally true.

For example, there was no action on the pupil and at no time was any increased salivation observed although no special experiments were done to check this point.

Furthermore, the undiminished activity after vagotomy, nicotine and atropine argue against a parasympathetic mediation. The action of the drug in causing contractions of virgin uteri regardless of the previous action of adrenalin on those uteri suggested a musculotropic action.

The assumption of musculotropic action means that the substance must act on smooth muscle in different locations in opposite fashion, that is, to relax the muscle of the vessel walls and constrict that of the uterus and intestine.

This seems unusual but it can be pointed out that synephrine and one or two other closely related sympathomimetic compounds have similar paradoxical actions and these drugs have been shown almost surely to be musculotropic.

# PASSION FLOWER & FRUIT: TOXIC RIDDLES FOR TOXIC DETECTIVE

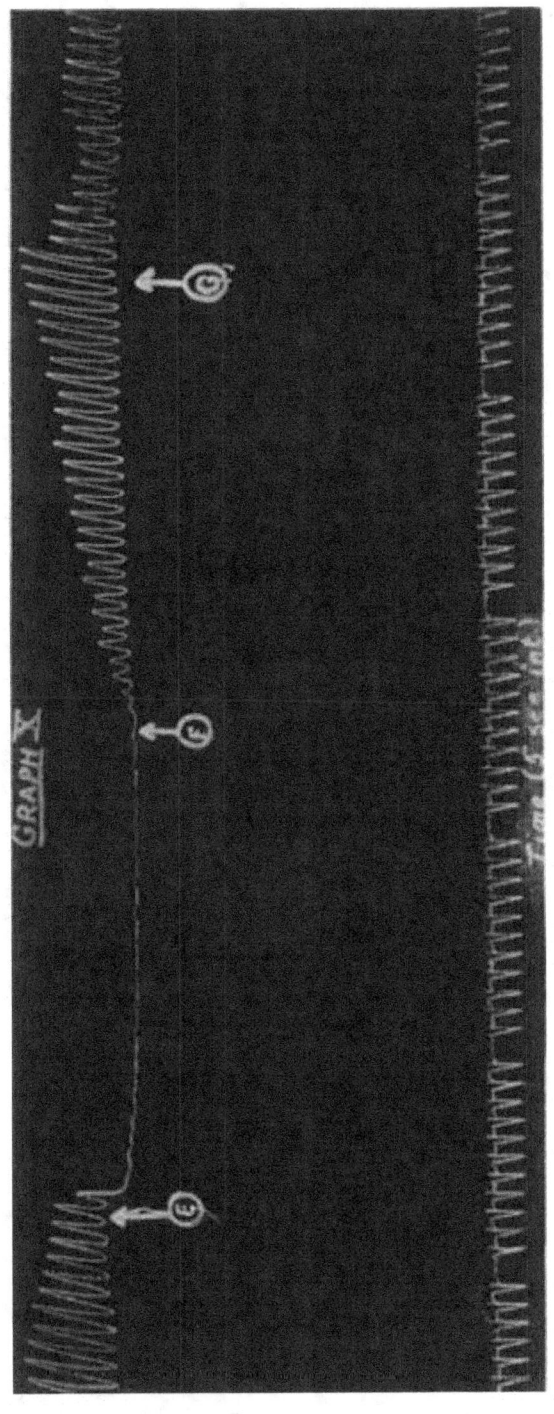

Figure 18. Isolated Intestinal Strip. Action of the Passiflora in Conjunction with Adrenalin. Source: Journal Of The American Pharmaceutical Association. Volume 29, Issue 6,1940, Pages 245-249.

The passiflora extract caused lowering of the blood pressure and contraction of smooth muscle of the gut and uterus.

The activity of the substance has been shown to be unaffected by vagotomy, atropine, nicotine or pituitrin.

The passiflora extract probably exerts its characteristic activity by direct action on smooth muscle.

Citation: George H. Ruggy, Clayton S. Smith. A pharmacological study of the active principle of passiflora incarnate. Journal Of The American Pharmaceutical Association. Volume 29, Issue 6,1940, Pages 245-249.

# MALT ALL, DRANK IN TEA FOR BAR

Malt all = malt-ol = maltol (homophonic)

Lyophilised hydroalcoholic and aqueous extracts of the aerial parts of Passiflora incarnata L. (Passifloraceae) (Passion-flower), as well as chemical constituents of the plant, indole alkaloids (harman, harmin, harmalin, harmol, and harmalol) maltol and flavonoids (orientin, isoorientin, vitexin and isovitexin) were assessed for behavioral effects in mice by Soulimani R, et al (1997).

To investigate the behavioural effects of P. incarnata extracts and its alkaloid and flavonoid derivatives and maltol, Soulimani R, et al. selected three behavioural tests allowing to investigate the psychotropic activity, specifically the sedative and anxiolytic properties: the staircase test, the light/dark box choice situation test—also known as constraint tests, and the free exploratory test—a non constraining test.

The results obtained have shown that the administration of an aqueous extract to mice induced a significant decrease of the number of rears. Then, the administration of a hydroalcoholic extract to mice induced a significant increase of the number of steps climbed. In comparison with results obtained after administration of hydroalcoholic extract at 400 mg/kg in the staircase test, the dose 800 mg/kg has not shown an anxiolytic-like activity. It appeared interesting to verify the effect of a dose of 800 mg/kg of hydroalcoholic extract on the free exploratory test which is specific for a sedative-like activity.

# STAIRCASE TEST

The involvement of some constituents of Passiflora incarnata L. such as indole alkaloid mixtures with maltol and flavonoid mixtures with maltol was examined, using the staircase test. Nor indole alkaloid mixtures with maltol, and none of the flavonoid mixtures with maltol modify any behavioural parameters in the staircase test.

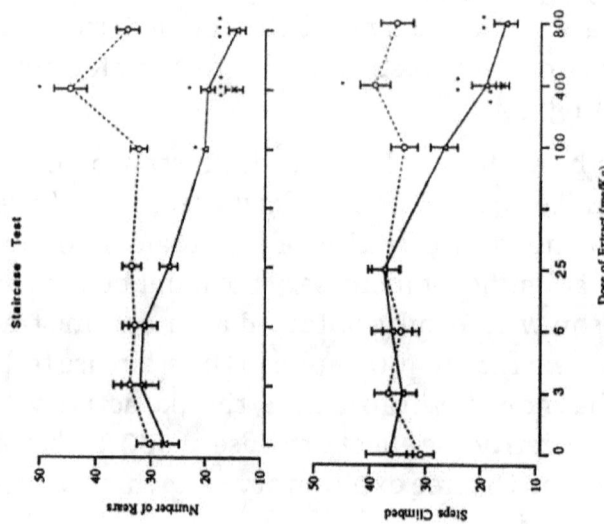

Figure 19. . Effect of aqueous and hydroalcoholic extract of Passiflora incarnata L. on the number of rears and steps climbed in the staircase test. Source: J Ethnopharmacol 1997;57:11–20.

# LIGHT /DARK TEST

The light/dark box choice situation test—corresponds to a constraining form of testing as the environment imposed to the animal implies an anxiety level that may cause behavioural inhibition, notably concerning the animal's exploratory, locomotor and motor activity.

This inhibitory effect may be suspended or cancelled by the administration of an anxiolytic substance.

The animal has the possibility of withdrawing from the light compartment to seek refuge in a dark one.

The administration of a hydroalcoholic extract induced a significant increase of the time spent and the number of rears in light side.

This effect was also observed in the staircase test at a dose of 400 mg/kg.

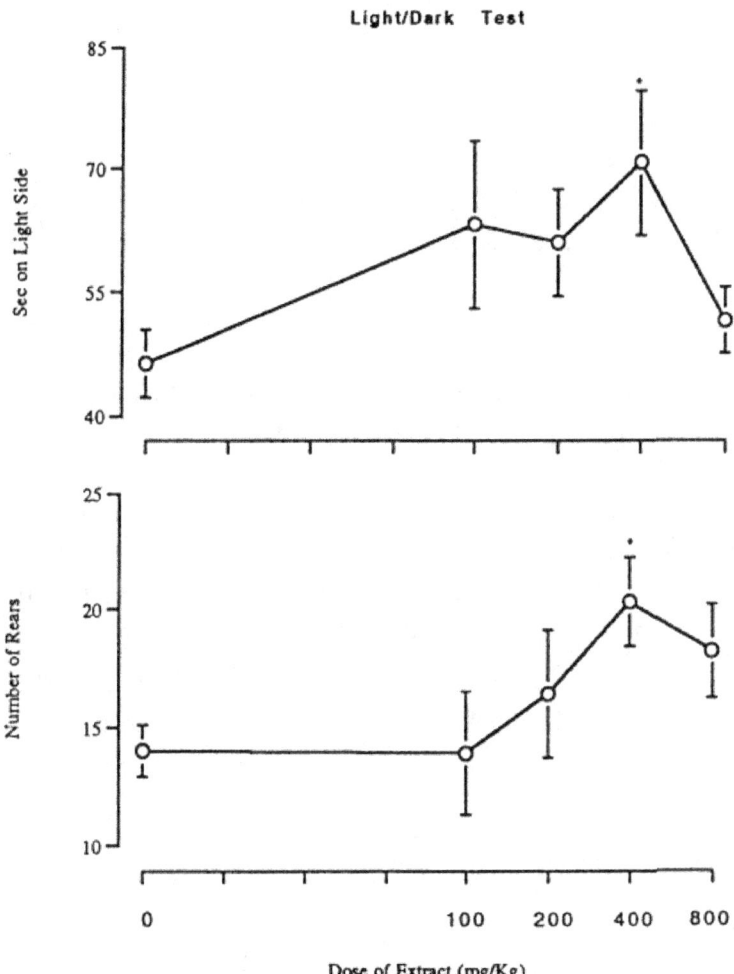

Figure 20. Effect of hydroalcoholic extract of Passiflora incarnata L. on the time spent in the light side and the number of rears in the light/dark test. Source: J Ethnopharmacol 1997;57:11–20.

And, the sleep-inducing action of these extracts in mice treated with a sub-hypnotic dose of sodium pentobarbital was investigated.

# FREE EXPLORATORY TEST

The free exploratory test offers a non-constraining and non-anxiogenic environment. This test has therefore some value to assess a sedative effect and can confirm the effect observed in the staircase test. The administration of an aqueous extract to mice induced a significant decrease of locomotion and the number of rears of mice submitted to a free exploratory test. This sedative effect observed in the staircase test was confirmed in the free exploratory test. It is dose-dependent in both cases, with a peak with 400 and 800 mg/kg doses.

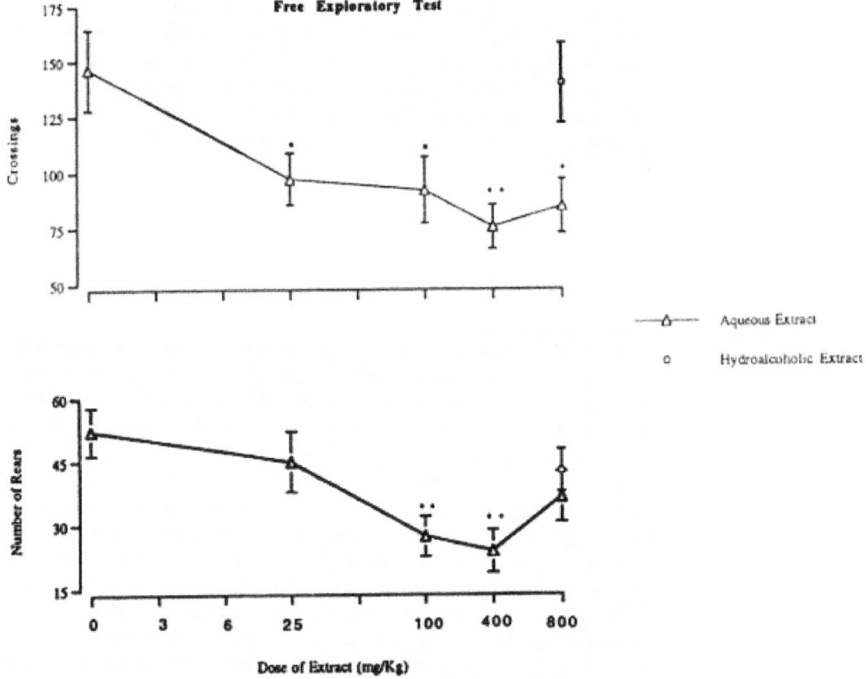

Figure 21.. Effect of aqueous and hydroalcoholic extract of Passiflora incarnata L. on the number of rears and crossings in the free exploratory test. Source: J Ethnopharmacol 1997;57:11-20.

On three tests, the aqueous extract appeared to induce sedative effects at 400 and 800 mg/kg.

It reduced activity in the staircase and free exploratory tests, as measured by the number of rears, steps climbed or locomotor crossings and potentiated the induction of sleeping by pentobarbital. Treatment with flumazenil (a benzodiazepine receptor antagonist) and the aqueous extract did not modify the activity in the staircase. The hydroalcoholic extract did not have such sedative effects. Instead, it appeared to enhance activity, suggestive of an anxiolytic effect at 400 mg/kg. Specifically, it increased the number of rears and steps climbed in the staircase test, and in the light/dark avoidance test it increased the time spent in the light compartment and the number of rears there.

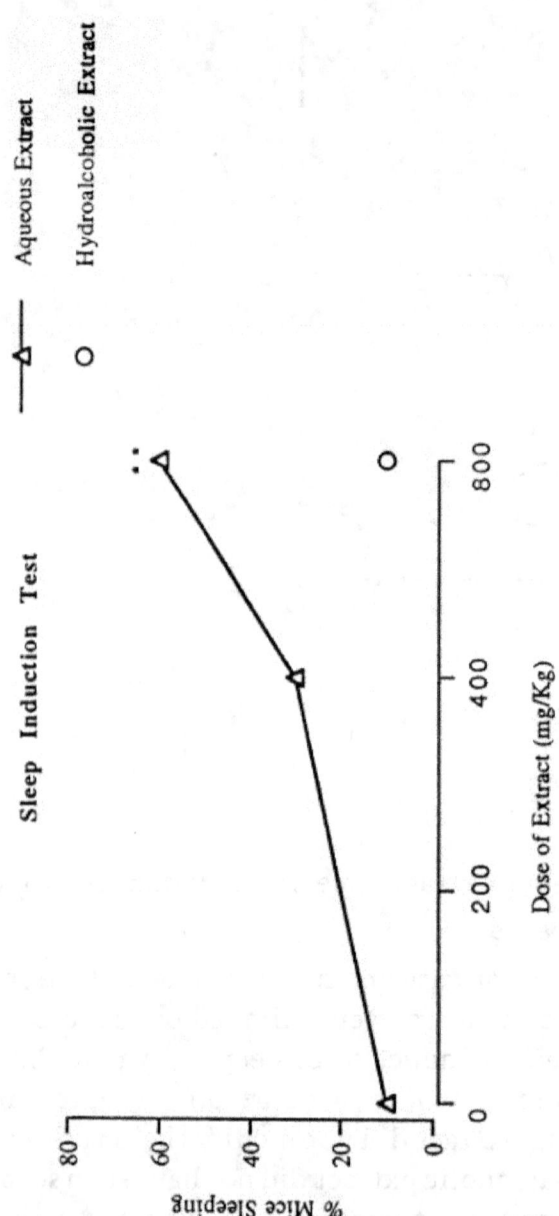

Figure 22. Effect of aqueous and hydroalcoholic extract of Passiflora incarnata L. on sleep induced by a sub-hypnotic dose of pentobarbital in mice; O indicates the group treated by saline (control). Source: J Ethnopharmacol 1997;57:11–20.

| | Harman (mg/kg) | Harmin (mg/kg) | Harmalin (mg/kg) | Harmol (mg/kg) | Harmalol (mg/kg) | Maltol (mg/kg) | DPM[a] (mg/kg) |
|---|---|---|---|---|---|---|---|
| A1 | 0.1 | 0.1 | 0.1 | 0.1 | 0.1 | 0.25 | 500 |
| A2 | 0.4 | 0.4 | 0.4 | 0.4 | 0.4 | 1 | 2000 |
| A3 | 1.6 | 1.6 | 1.6 | 1.6 | 1.6 | 4 | 8000 |
| A4 | 3.6 | 3.6 | 3.6 | 3.6 | 3.6 | 9 | 18 000 |

Indole alkaloids and maltol doses administred i.p. in mice

[a] Doses expressed in terms of dry plant material.
A. Mixture of alkaloids.

Figure 23. Indole alkaloids and maltol doses administred i.p. in mice. Source: J Ethnopharmacol 1997;57:11–20.

Citation: Soulimani R, et al. Behavioral effects of Passiflora incarnata L. and its indole alkaloid and flavonoid derivatives and maltol in the mouse. J Ethnopharmacol 1997;57:11–20.

# PASSIFLORINE

One of the six alkaloids has been listed as "passiflorine."

It has been called the active principle of P. incarnata by some herbalists.

Other researchers have not referred to it at all.

The Agricultural Research Service (ARS) Web site describes passiflorine as having no activity.

Citation: Agricultural Research Service Web site. Online document at: www.ars-grin.gov/duke/

A search of the Chemical Abstract Service's database under the search term "passiflorine" brings up a com- pound with the name passiflorin.

This is a steroid-like molecule, a derivative of 1H,19H-Cyclopropa[9,10]cyclopenta[a]phenanthrene, 9,19-cycloergostane-4-carboxylic acid.

It has been identified as a component of P. edulis leaves and stems.

Citation: Yoshikawa, K. et al. Four cycloartane triterpenoids and six related saponins from Passiflora edulis. J Nat Prod 2000;63:1229–1234.

It would not produce a positive result on an alkaloid test as has been reported for the compound "passiflorine" in one analysis of P. incarnata.

Citation: Online document at: www.passionflower.org/

passionanalysis.html

### Passiflorin

Passiflorin is obviously not related to harmane.

No investigations into passiflorin's bioactivity have been reported nor has it been identified as a synonym for "passiflorine" as yet.

Citation: Cronin JR. 2003. Passionflower Reigniting male libido and other potential uses. Altern Complement Ther 9 89–92.

# CHEMICAL ANALYSIS

The composition of Passiflora's phytochemical content is not well-established.

There have been several studies of the alkaloids, flavonoids, and their glycoside and glycosyl derivatives in Passiflora plants but many of these studies disagree on the compounds that are present in P. incarnate.

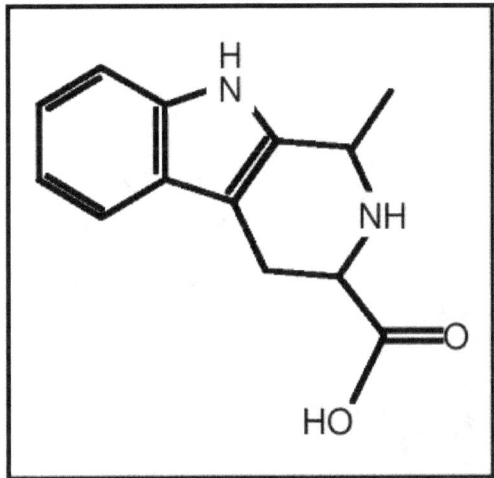

Figure 24. Harmane as indole alkaloid in Passiflora: Chemical structure

# ELECTROPHORESIS

Electrophoresis of the plant extracts permitted the identification of at least four protein bands for passion flower. The passion flower extract submitted to electrophoresis was separated into several protein bands of molecular weight ranging from 20.1 to 94 kD.

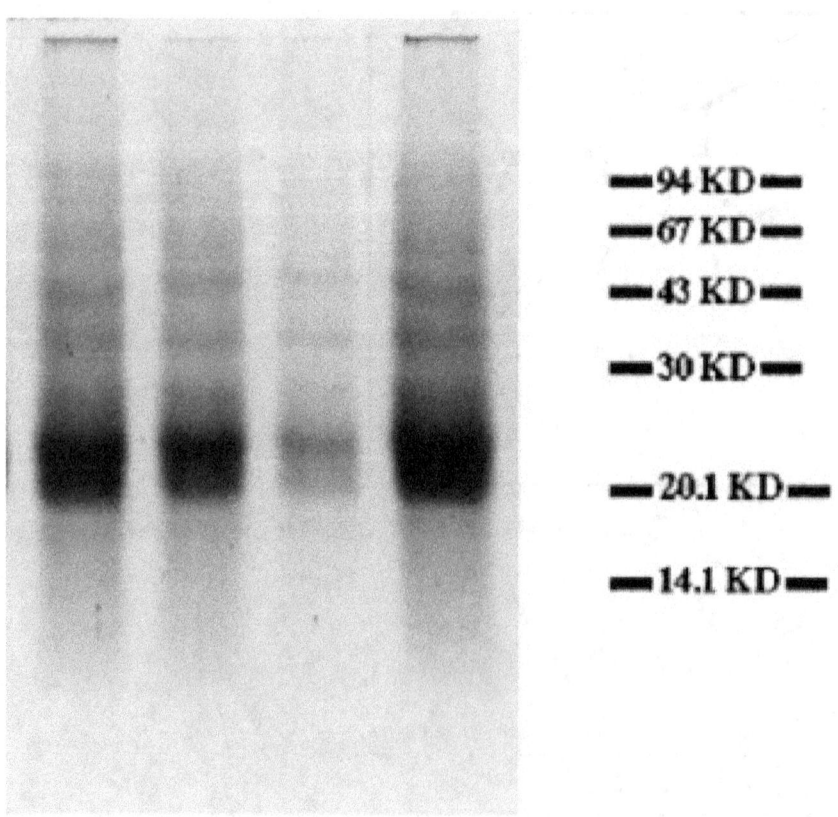

Figure 25. Electrophoresis of passion flower. Source: Ann Allergy Asthma Im-

munol 1997;79:449–454.

The ethnobotanical database on the U.S. Agricultural Research Service's Web site lists the total alkaloid content of P. incarnata as 100 to 900 ppm and the total flavonoid content as 1.2–3.9 percent.

Some active principles have been isolated from the plant using thin layer chromatography (TLC). Harman, harmine, and harmol have been extracted from the alkaloid phase, and vitexin, iso-vitexin, orientin, iso-orientin, and saponarin from the flavonoid phase.

# WESTERN BLOTTING

Western blotting confirmed in vitro the sensitization of the patient to a protein of approximately 20 kD of passion flower.

The Western blot technique revealed IgE and IgG antibodies in the patient's serum against a protein of approximately 20-kD molecular weight present in the passion flower extract.

On the tape with control serum there was no IgE antibody binding, but IgG antibody binding to a protein band of approximately 35 kD did occur.

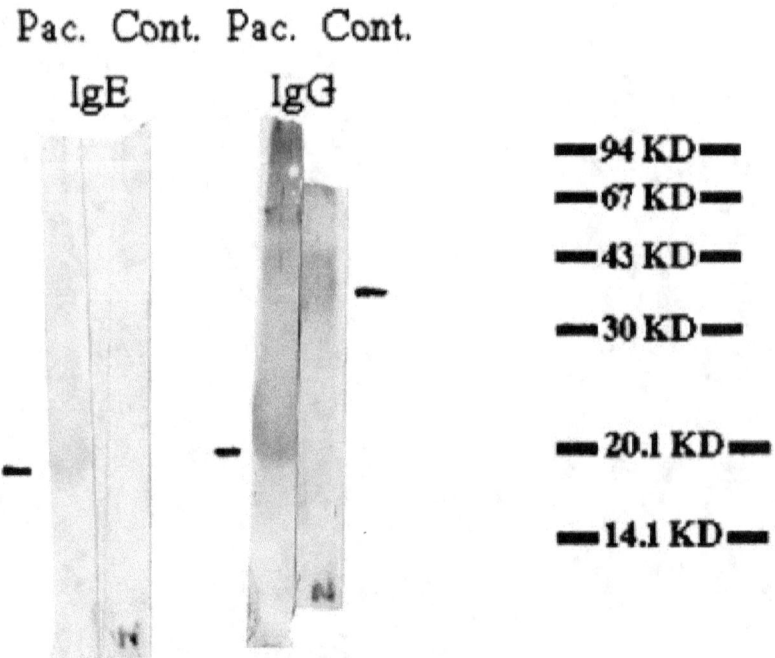

Figure 26. Western blot analysis of passion flower. Source: Ann Allergy Asthma Immunol 1997;79:449–454.

Twenty-six components fall into two categories: 20 flavonoids (including a cyanogenic glycoside and gynocardine) and 6 alkaloids.

**List of Flavonoids**

| Compound | R3 | R5 | R6 | R7 | R8 | R1' | R2' | R3' | R4' | R5' |
|---|---|---|---|---|---|---|---|---|---|---|
| Flavone | H | H | H | H | H | H | H | H | H | H |
| Apigenin | H | OH | H | OH | H | H | H | OH | H | H |
| Luteolin | H | OH | H | OH | H | H | OH | OH | H | H |
| Chrysin | MeO | OH | H | OH | H | H | OH | MeO | H | H |

MeO = Methoxy.

# MARACUJA

The Portuguese name Maracuja has been applied to both P. incarnata and P. edulis.

They are, however, distinct species.

P edulis or yellow passionflower is the plant that provides the familiar, edible passion fruit.

Other confusion arises from the species name Passiflora alata.

The Alternative Medicine Foundations Web site HerbMed lists P. alata, as the species name for "passion flower," but the literature references found on the site refer to research done on P. incarnata.

The botanical database of United States Department of Agriculture (USDA) lists the two as separate species.

P. incarnata (botanical symbol PAIN6) is listed as a species native to the United States with distribution through 18 southern and southeastern states.

P. alata (botanical symbol PAAL27) is listed as "non-native or cultivated."

The USDA site also gives the common name "passion flower" to P. alata and "purple passion flower" to P. incarnata.

Additional confusion arises in considering the active chemical components of the various species.

# DECODING

Harm in Pass I, on vine

= Harm in= Harmine

=Pass I, on vine= paasion vine

Other Names: Apricot vine, Granadilla, Maypop, Passion vine

hamaline, harmalol, harmine and harmol

Passionflower contains several flavonoids (apigenin, benzoflavone and others), harmala alkaloids (hamaline, harmalol, harmine and harmol), coumarins, maltol, phytosterols and glycosides.

Recent Studies in laboratory animals suggest that extracts of passionflower have sedative, anxiolytic, analgesic and antispasmodic effects.

Although passionflower extracts are classified as "Generally Regarded as Safe" by the FDA, there have been some case reports of adverse reactions.

# ALLERGY

One case of occupational allergic reaction induced by Passiflora alata, has also been reported by Giavina-Bianchi PF, et al (1997).

Work in a pharmacy for the manual preparation of medications, a quite common activity in Brazil, with inhalation of various substances of high molecular weight, may be considered a condition extremely favorable to the development of diseases of the airways due to hypersensitivity.

Case Report: The patient had been working for 2 years in a pharmacy devoted to the manual preparation of products, where he weighed and prepared chemical products eight hours each day, Monday through Saturday, without using a mask, gloves, or other protective materials. In mid-1992, when he had been working at the pharmacy for 6 months, the patient started to experience episodes of sneezing, coryza, and nasal pruritus and congestion. He also reported ocular pruritus and hyperemia, tearing, and pruritus of the auditory canal and oropharynx. Three months after the original symptoms, he developed a dry cough, chest pain, sensations of chest tightening, dyspnea, and wheezing. The symptoms started to be continuous and were worse in the morning when he entered the pharmacy, and when he manipulated capsules containing passion flower preparations. The symptoms improved after the end of the working day, but on some occasions worsened again at night in his house. There was also relief of symptoms on Sundays. The patient had been using inhaled 2-adrenergic agents frequently. He had no history of atopy but had a smoking habit of 1 pack per day of 16 years' duration. Physical examination revealed that the nasal turbinates were slightly hypertrophied and hyperemic. The patient had a respiratory rate of 20 rpm without using accessory respiratory muscles, with moderate wheezing heard diffusely on both sides of the chest upon auscultation. The peak expiratory flow rate was 480 L/minute (predicted: 622). Laboratory tests showed 14% eosinophilia with 8,000 leukocytes per cubic min and total IgE levels of 1130 IU/mL. The pulmonary function test suggested moderate bronchial obstruction with no significant reversibility after the use of appropriate medication (FVC: 71%; FEV1: 68%; FEV/FCV ratio: 97%; FEF25–75%: 47%; PFR: 73%). The patient was advised to leave his job until he could be better studied. He began to use 1000 g of beclomethasone per day.

The existence of a "period of latency of exposure", i.e., a period of 6 months from the beginning of exposure to the drugs to the onset of symptoms, suggests an IgE-mediated disease.

Skin testing and Western blot confirmed the sensitization of the patient to these plant extracts in vivo and in vitro, respectively.

Bronchial challenge confirmed the cause-effect relationship between the allergen exposure and the diseases.

Passiflora is new etiologic agent of IgE-mediated occupational asthma and rhinitis.

This study also serves to alert physicians to the risks associated with work in pharmacies devoted to manual preparation of plant extracts, emphasizing the importance of the use of protective measures in these environments.

| CONTROL | | HISTAMINE (10 mg/ml) |
|---|---|---|
| | | ●     ⎯ 1 cm |
| CONCENTRATION [1] | PASSIONFLOWER [2] | CASCARA SAGRADA [3] |
| 0.01% | ● | ● |
| 0.1% | ● | ● |
| 1% | ● | ● |
| 10% | ● | ● |

Figure 27. sizes of the wheals observed in the prick tests with passion flower. Source: Ann Allergy Asthma Immunol 1997;79:449–454.

The first challenge with histamine indicated bronchial hyperreactivity, with a PC20 of 0.150 mg/mL, although the patient had left his working environment 9 months earlier and was using beclomethasone by inhalation.

The observation of a variation in FEV1 on the day of challenge with physiologic saline is compatible with the known fact that the higher the hyperreactivity of the bronchial tree, the greater the variation of daily pulmonary function.

Specific bronchial challenge demonstrated that the patient experienced acute asthma after allergen inhalation, with a significant reduction of FEV1 compared with basal values, i.e., an

18.75% reduction with the inhalation of 0.0024 mg passion flower.

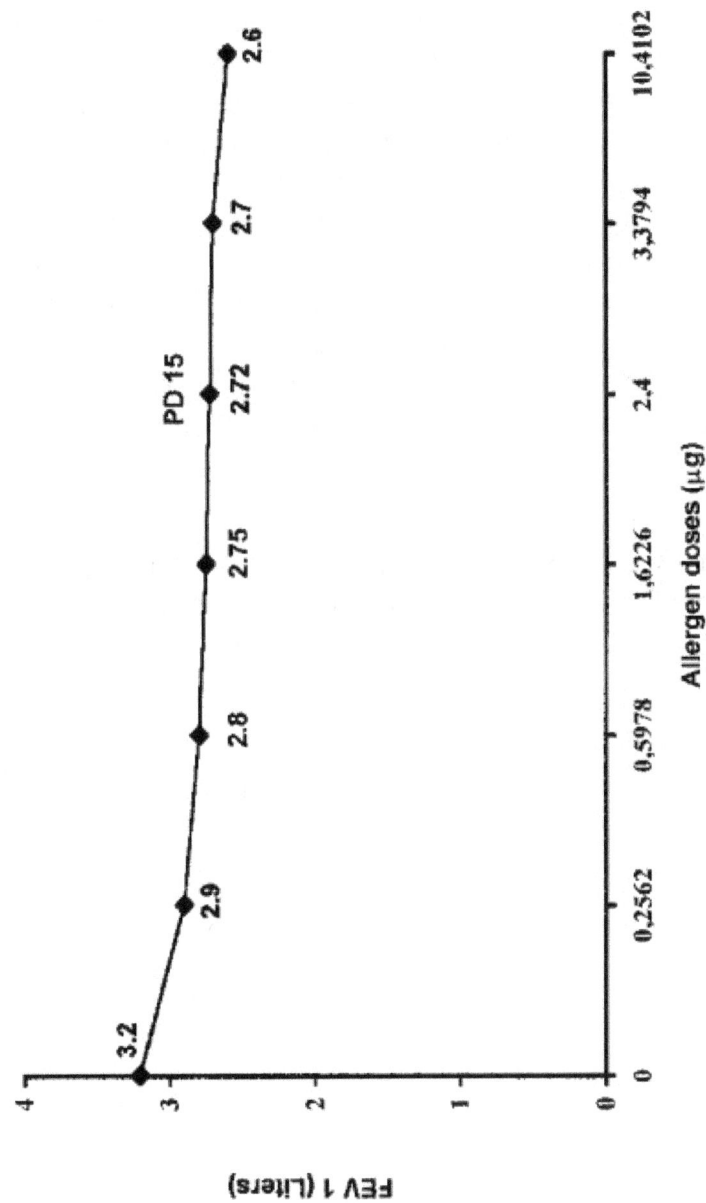

Figure 28. FEV1 measured after the inhalation by the patient of different doses of passion flower. Ann Allergy Asthma Immunol 1997;79:449–454.

There are three clues indicating that the bronchoconstriction triggered by the plant extracts was due to a mechanism of type I hypersensitivity. First, and most important, control individuals, including asthmatic patients with bronchial hyperreactivity, did not have positive tests even when they inhaled a 1% allergen solution. Second, the occurrence of delayed symptoms, with a 43.75% fall in basal FEV1 upon challenge with passion flower and a 26.31% fall upon challenge with cascara sagrada, suggests an IgE-mediated allergic response. Last, the second challenge with histamine, performed after the specific challenge, showed that the airway was more constricted, more reactive, and possibly more inflamed due to allergen exposure than on the occasion of the first examination carried out before challenge with the allergens.

Giavina-Bianchi PF, et al. Occupational respiratory allergic disease induced by Passiflora alata and Rhamnus purshiana. Ann Allergy Asthma Immunol 1997;79:449–454.

# LIVER TOXICITY BY PASSION

The ARS Web site reports lethal and toxic doses of dry and alcoholic extract of Passionflower as:

$LD_{50}$ = 3000–15,000 mg/kg;

Toxic dose = 500–900 mg/kg.

LiverTox: Clinical and Research Information on Drug-Induced Liver Injury [Internet]. Bethesda (MD): National Institute of Diabetes and Digestive and Kidney Diseases; 2012-. Passionflower. [Updated 2020 Mar 28]. Available from: https://www.ncbi.nlm.nih.gov/books/NBK548020/

# PASSIO= SUFFER

Pass see-flow-raw= Pas-si-flo-ra

Passiflora Passion-flower, (patior, pati, passus)-florum (the signature of the numbers of parts in the flower related to the events of the Passion) (Passifloraceae) passionis -is -e of Passion-tide, late Latin passio (in the sense of suffering).

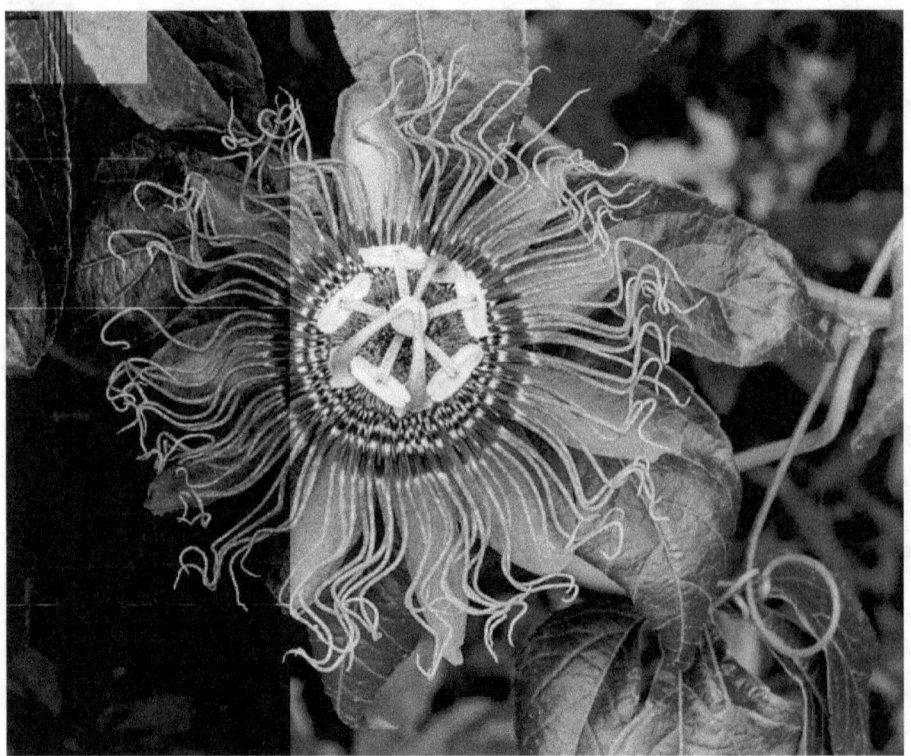

Figure 29. Passiflora incarnata, Passion Vine, purple petals and purple corona filaments variety, at the Butterfly Garden at Norfolk Botanical Garden, Norfolk, Virginia. PumpkinSky (2017)wikipedia.

# DOSAGE RECOMMENDATIONS

Therapeutic dose recommendations range between 2 and 8 g of a dry extract equivalent per day, with the maximum amount corresponding to a dose of 100 mg/kg per day for an average adult.

Ref: Duke JA, ed. CRC Handbook of Medicinal Herbs. Boca Raton, FL: CRCPress, 1985.

# CONFUSION IN ITS EFFICACY

Because the active principals of the plants are not yet well characterized, and, because there are some differences in the reported chemical analyses of Passiflora plants, there is good reason to be wary of their medicinal product sources.

A recent study by Dhawan K, et al (2002) of the anxiolytic effects of the plant extract on laboratory mice compared a standardized preparation of a P. incarnata extract with several commercially available extracts supplied by what the study authors described as "reputable companies."

There were differences between the efficacies of the commercial products and the standardized preparation. One of the commercial products produced no anxiolytic effect at all.

Their report suggested that, in addition to shelf-life issues, there could easily be **confusion** regarding the manufacturers' plant supplies because of the similarities of the species P. incarnata and P. edulis.

ANTIANXIETY EFFECTS OF THE MARKETED MOTHER TINCTURES OF *PASSIFLORA INCARNATA* AT FOUR DOSES, 45 MINUTES AFTER ORAL ADMINISTRATION

| Company that marketed mother tincture | Dose mg/kg | Mean time spent in open arms ± SD |
|---|---|---|
| SBL Ltd. | 100 | 2.8 ± 0.45[a] |
| | 200 | 8.6 ± 1.95[a] |
| | **300** | **36.6 ± 4.98**[b] |
| | 400 | 7.4 ± 2.88[a] |
| Dr. Willmar Schwabe, Germany | 100 | 4.2 ± 0.84[a] |
| | 200 | 3.6 ± 0.89[a] |
| | 300 | 14.2 ± 4.21[a] |
| | **400** | **35.2 ± 4.55**[b] |
| Dr. Willmar Schwabe, India | 100 | 3.7 ± 1.48[a] |
| | 200 | 6.4 ± 1.67[a] |
| | 300 | 7.2 ± 1.10[a] |
| | **400** | **35.6 ± 4.93**[b] |
| Dr. Reckeweg & Co. | 100 | — |
| | **200** | **38.8 ± 5.31**[b] |
| | 300 | 16.8 ± 2.68[a] |
| | 400 | — |
| Bhandari Homoeopathic Lab. | 100 | — |
| | 200 | 2.2 ± 0.45[a] |
| | 300 | — |
| | 400 | — |
| Standard (bioactive dose of methanol extract of *P. incarnata*) | 125 | 40.4 ± 5.61 |
| Control | 0.25 mL | — |

[a]Significantly more than the value of control but significantly different from standard.
[b]Significantly more than the value of control but insignificantly different with respect to standard.
Value expressed as mean ± SD; $n = 5$; $P < 0.05$ vs. control and standard, ANOVA followed by Fischer's least significantly different test.
SD, standard deviation; ANOVA, analysis of variance. Bold type indicates the highest possible anxiolytic dose.

Figure 30. anxiolytic activity profiles of various marketed mother tinctures of Passiflora incarnata. **Source:** The Journal Of Alternative And Complementary Medicine. Volume 8, Number 3, 2002, pp. 283–291

Dhawan K, et al. Comparative anxiolytic activity profile of various preparations of Passiflora incarnata Linneaus: A comment on medicinal plants' standardization. J Altern Complement Med 2002;8:283–291.

# THE ACHE BUILDS IN TUMMY FOR

HUG TEARS STAINED PILLOW CLOSE
WHEN NO ONE IS ANYWAY AROUND
AND CRIES FOR ONE U LOVED & LOST
AND SCREAMS WITHOUT A SOUND
OTHERS SEE YOU IN A BRIGHT DAY
AND THINKS YOU ARE DOING WELL
BUT EVERY DAY AS EVENING SETS
I SEE YOU ENTER YOUR OWN HELL
TIME HASN'T HEALED U AT ALL
OR QUIETED YOUR OWN FEARS

This above rhyming poem described the repeating story of Drug abusers, especially opium addicts, who suffer from insomnia, in absence of opium abuse, craving & crying in pain silently, in their beds, holding their tummies.

# PASSION FOR MORPHINE

In the traditional system of medicine in India, Passiflora incarnata Linn. (Passifloraceae; synonyms: passionflower, maracuja, maypops, Krishan-Kamala) attracted our attention due to various reports regarding the use of the plant in breaking down the morphine habit in addicts.

A fraction (BZF) derived from the methanol extract of P. incarnata that had exhibited good anxiolytic activity, delayed the development of tolerance to the analgesic effect of morphine when administered at 10, 50 and 100 mg/kg doses along with 10 mg/kg dose of morphine for 9 days.

A single dose of P. incarnata bioactive fraction (BZF) also decreased the naloxone precipitated withdrawal jumps in mice that had already been rendered tolerant due to chronic treatment with 10 mg/kg of morphine.

Citation: Dhawan, et al. Reversal of Morphine Tolerance and Dependence by Passiflora incarnata – A Traditional Medicine to Combat Morphine Addiction. Pharmaceutical Biology. 40:8, 576-580, DOI: 10.1076/phbi.40.8.576.14660

# RX OPIATE ADDICTS

Accumulating evidence shows the efficacy of Passiflora incarnata extract in the management of opioid addiction related anxiety, so may be used as an adjuvant agent in the detoxification of opiates by clonidine & oxazepam.

The main disadvantage of clonidine-based detoxification, in addition to a hypotensive effect, is lack of efficacy for mental symptoms.

Benzodiazepines are not recommended, as they may induce dependence.

There is increasing evidence that extracts of Passiflora incarnata have sedative-hypnotic and anxiolytic properties without inducing dependence.

Citation: Bergner P. (1995) Passionflower. Medical Herbalism, 7, 13±14, 26.

Two studies on opium addicts were done by team of psychiatrists (Akhondzadeh S, et al) using clonidine & oxazepam along with passiflora, in two separate groups in the same year(2001), in same Hospital (Roozbeh Psychiatric Hospital, Tehran University of Medical Sciences, South Kargar Avenue, Tehran) as double-blind randomized controlled trial.

The main overall findings from these studies are:

(i) that both treatments reduce physical symptoms of acute opiate withdrawal syndrome but the passiflora-clonidine combination may have a more rapid onset of action, and

(ii) that passiflora extract may be of therapeutic benefit in the management of mental symptoms of opiate withdrawal.

First study by Akhondzadeh S, et al (2001) examined the use of P. incarnata extract in conjunction with clonidine for treating patients who are addicted to opium for withdrawal symptoms.

| Short Opiate Withdrawal Scale (SOWS) |
|---|
| • Feeling sick<br>• Stomach cramps<br>• Muscle spasm/ twitching<br>• Feeling of coldness<br>• Heart pounding<br>• Muscle tension<br>• Aches and pains<br>• Yawning<br>• Runny eyes<br>• Insomnia/problems sleeping<br>• Diarrhoea<br>• Dysphoria<br>• Anxiety<br>• Agitation<br>• Irritability<br>• Craving for substances |

The mean ‹ SEM scores for the two groups are shown in Figure below. There were no significant differences in baseline mental symptoms between the two treatment groups. A RM-ANOVA showed a significant effect with both treatments on the mental symptoms scores. Post-hoc testing revealed a significant reduction from baseline in the passiflora group from day 2, but not in the clonidine group. The mean mental scores for the clonidine group were significantly higher than for the passiflora group on days 2, 3, 4, 7 and 14.

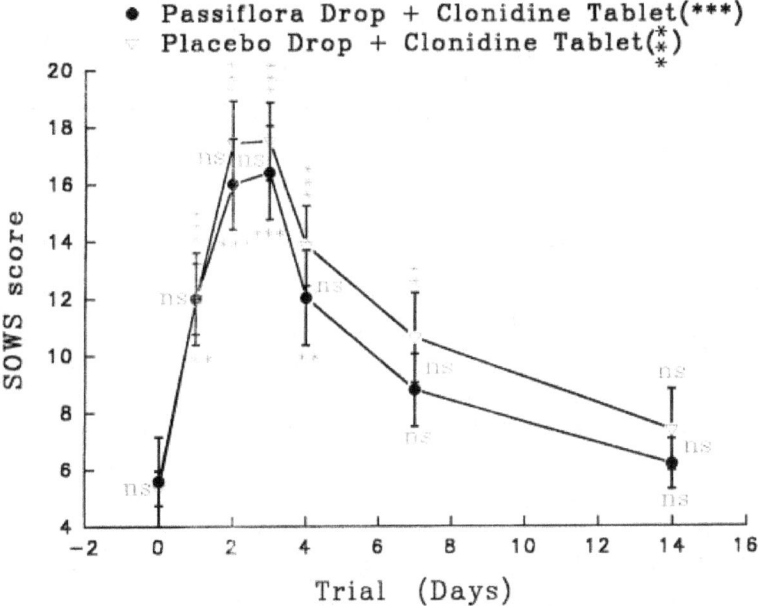

Figure 31. Short Opiate Withdrawal Scale(SOWS) with Passiflora & clonidine. Source: J Clin Pharm Ther 2001;26:369-373.

The report compared the combination treatment with the clonidine plus placebo treatment of 65 subjects suffering from withdrawal from a variety of opiates.

The study revealed no significant difference in the effects of the two regimens on physical symptoms (e.g., aching, nausea, cramps, etc.).

The researchers did report that subjects who were treated with the P. incarnata/clonidine combination were able to manage their mental symptoms (anxiety, irritability, craving etc.) better.

There was no description of the P. incarnata extract used.

Akhondzadeh S, et al. Passionflower in the treatment of opiate withdrawal: A double blind randomized controlled trial. J Clin Pharm Ther 2001;26:369-373.

The second study by Akhondzadeh S, et al (2001) described the treatment of 36 patients with generalized anxiety disorder. Treatment with oxazepam plus a placebo dose of liquid (group 1) was compared to liquid treatment with a P. incarnata extract plus a placebo tablet (group 2).

The patients in group 1 had lower anxiety scores than the patients in group 2 during the first 15 days of treatment. After this period, there were no significant differences between the two groups.

A comparison of side-effects in the two groups showed no significant differences, apart from a higher incidence of job performance impairment in the oxazepam-treated group.

Akhondzadeh A. et al. Passionflower in the treatment of generalized anxiety: A pilot double-blind randomized controlled trial with oxazepam. J Clin Pharm Ther 2001;26:363–367.

# RESTORATION SEXUALITY

Dhawan K, Sharma A. Restoration of chronic- Delta(9)-THC-induced decline in sexuality in male rats by a novel benzoflavone moiety from Passiflora incarnata Linn. Br J Pharmacol 2003;138:117–120.

# SIDE EFFECTS

Altered consciousness

Loss of coordination

Confusion

Dizziness

Drowsiness

Liver toxicity

Nausea/vomiting

Liver & Pancreas toxicity

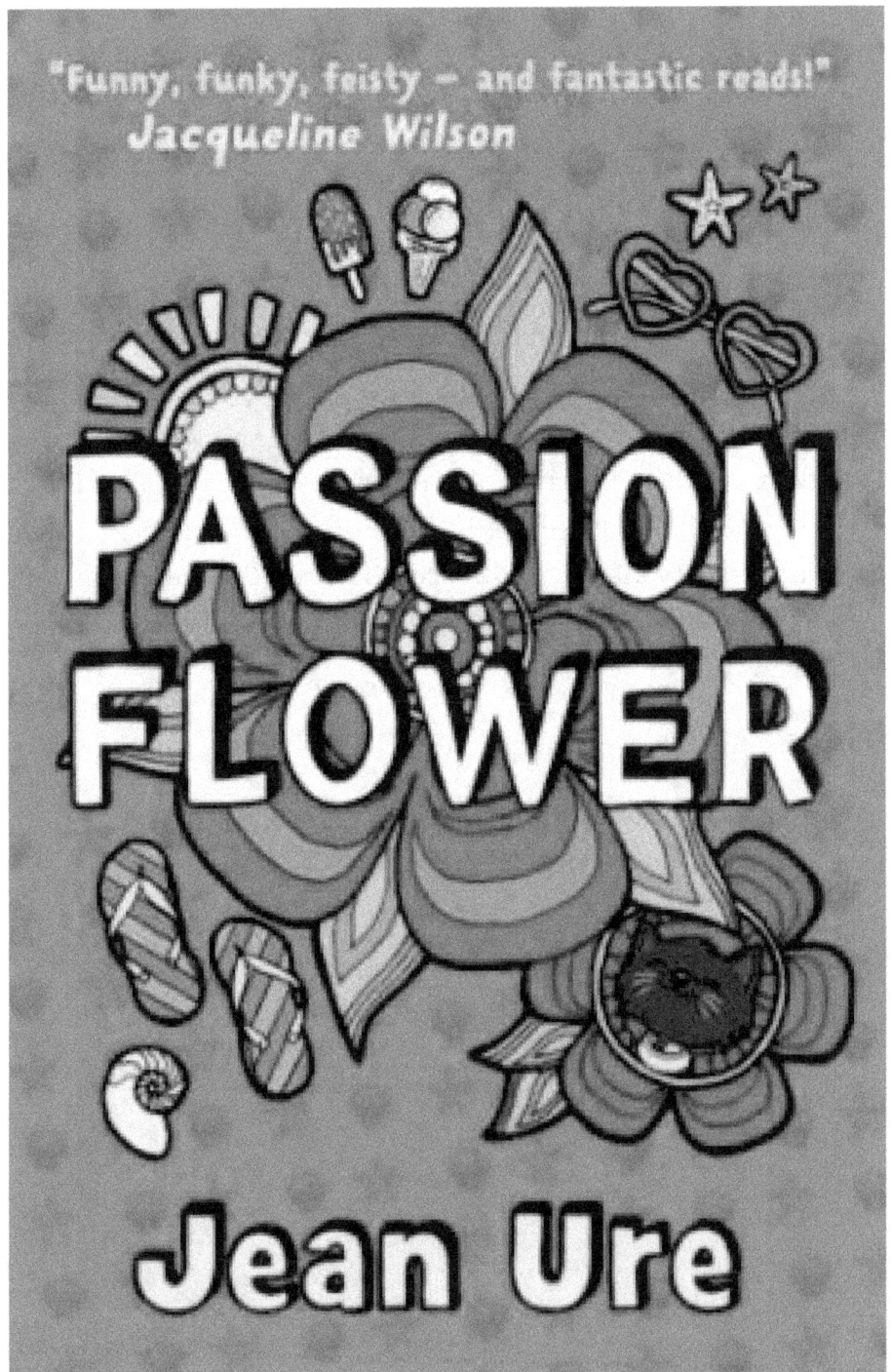

# IS PASSIFLORA CAERULEA POISONOUS?

Passiflora caerulea is harmful if ingested and causes an upset stomach. Its foliage and roots are toxic.

Citation: Bradley PR, ed. (1992) British Herbal Compendium, Vol. 1. Bournemouth: British Herbal Medicine Association.

# CAN PASSIONFLOWER CAUSE LIVER DAMAGE?

Passionflower has not been implicated in causing serum enzyme elevations or clinically apparent liver injury.

# TOXICITY MAY POP, TO LIVE, ARE

May Pop = In May, Passion flower pops out

Live-are = live-R (homophonic)

Toxicity may pop up by Passiflora incarnate.

Fisher AA et al (2000) reported that a 34-year-old female developed severe nausea, vomiting, drowsiness, prolonged QTc, and episodes of nonsustained ventricular tachycardia following self-administration of a herbal remedy, Passiflora incarnata L., at therapeutic doses.

The possible association of symptoms with passiflora was not recognized for several days.

She required hospital admission for cardiac monitoring and intravenous fluid therapy.

It is important to ask specifically about the use of herbal medicines in patients with undiagnosed illnesses.

Herbal medicines may have significant adverse effects which are not suspected or recognized.

Citation: Fisher AA, Purcell P, et al. Toxicity of Passiflora incarnata L. J Toxicol Clin Toxicol. 2000;38(1):63-66.

# DOES PASSION FLOWER INCREASE SEROTONIN?

In animals, passionflower is known to enhance spatial memory and reduce stress while decreasing serotonin levels. In a study done on humans, passionflower has been shown to remedy minor sleep problems in adults after a week.

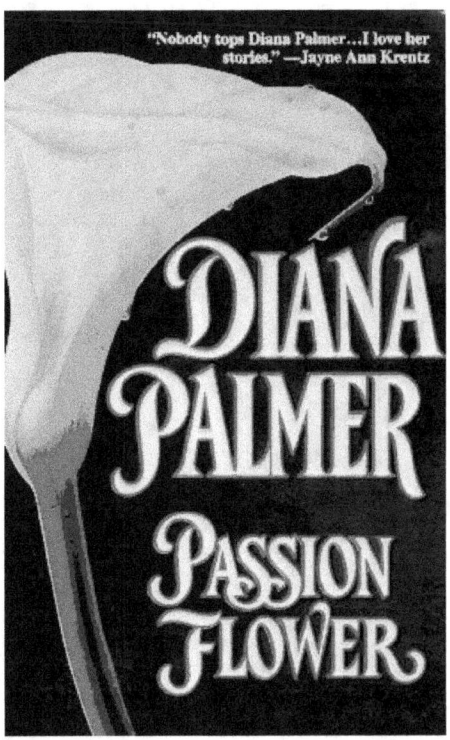

Figure 32. Passion Flower. Diana Palmer 1996.

# DOES IT MAKE YOU SLEEPY?

Passionflower might cause sleepiness and drowsiness. Medications that cause sleepiness are called sedatives. Taking passionflower along with sedative medications might cause too much sleepiness.

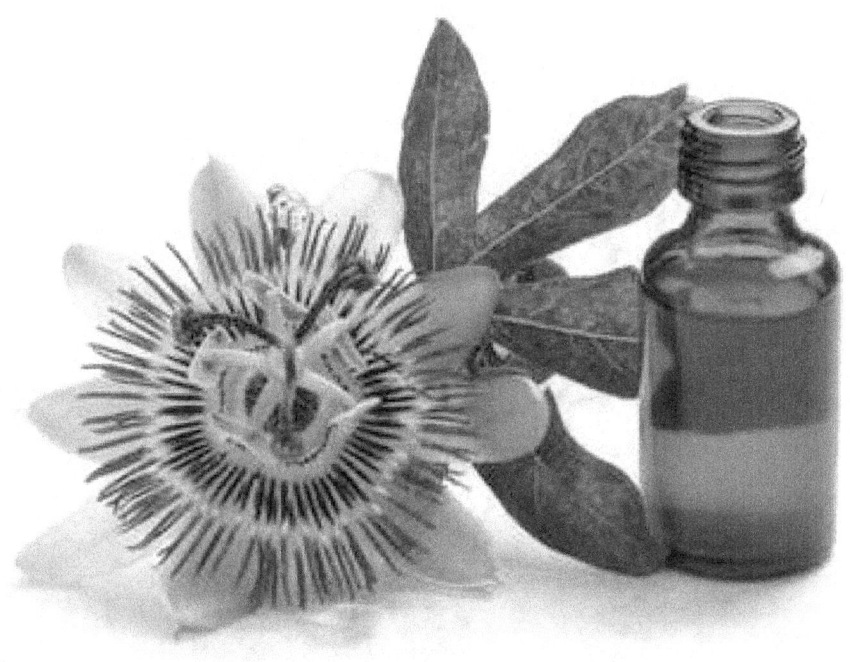

# IS IT ADDICTIVE?

Passion flower is thought to induce sleep, aid in reducing anxiety, help with relaxation, and aid those suffering from addiction with withdrawal symptoms.

In clinical studies, passiflora has been compared to other anxiety medications such as oxazepam.

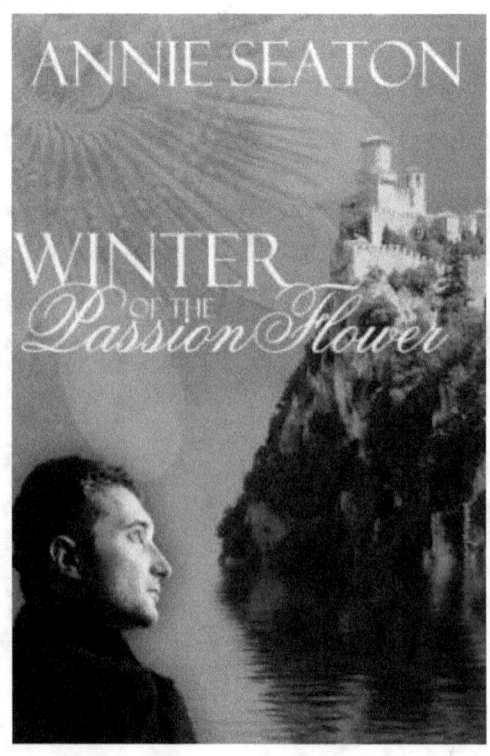

Figure 33. Winter of the Passion Flower. Seaton Annie. Year:2012

# WHAT IS PASSIFLORA USED FOR?

For example, Passiflora incarnata may help treat anxiety and insomnia.

Native Americans have used passionflower to treat a variety of conditions.

These include boils, wounds, earaches, and liver problems.

There are many different species of passion flower, but the one used for its medicinal benefits is Passiflora incarnate.

It goes by other names like maypop and wild apricot and is the state wildflower of Tennessee.

# DOES PASSION FLOWER INTERACT WITH ANYTHING?

Passionflower may interact with the following medications: Sedatives (drugs that cause sleepiness) -- Because of its calming effect, passionflower may increase the effects of sedative medications. These can include: Anticonvulsants such as phenytoin (Dilantin).

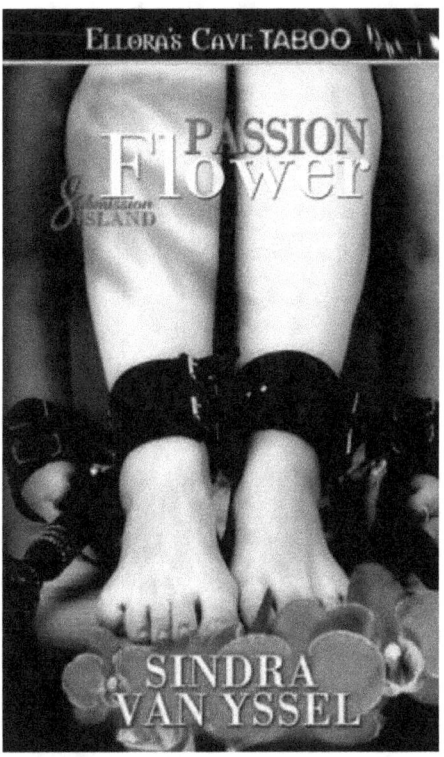

Figure 34 Passion Flower. Yssel Sindra van. Year:2013

# REIGNITING MALE LIBIDO

Benzoflavone's ability to restore reduced libido in aging male rats, restore fertility and libido by passiflora extract.

Cronin JR. 2003. Passionflower: Reigniting male libido and other potential uses. Altern Complement Ther 9: 89–92.

Passiflora restore fertility and libido that has been reduced by alcohol or nicotine use.

Dhawan K, Sharma A. Prevention of chronic alcohol and nicotineinduced azospermia, sterility and decreased libido, by a novel tri-substituted benzoflavone moiety from Passiflora incarnata Linneaus in healthy male rats. Life Sci 2002;71:3059–3069

# DO PASSION FLOWERS SMELL?

Passiflora foetida. Passion flowers are some of nature's most strikingly beautiful flowers, and this one is no exception! ... Beyond its beautiful flower, this species is easy to recognize in the field by its disagreeable odor when disturbed.

# WHAT IS THE HARDIEST PASSION FLOWER?

Three-inch wide, creamy pink petals in a fully banded corolla appear throughout the summer. This is the hardiest of the Passion Flowers growing as far north as New England.

Maypop Passion Flower (Passiflora incarnata).

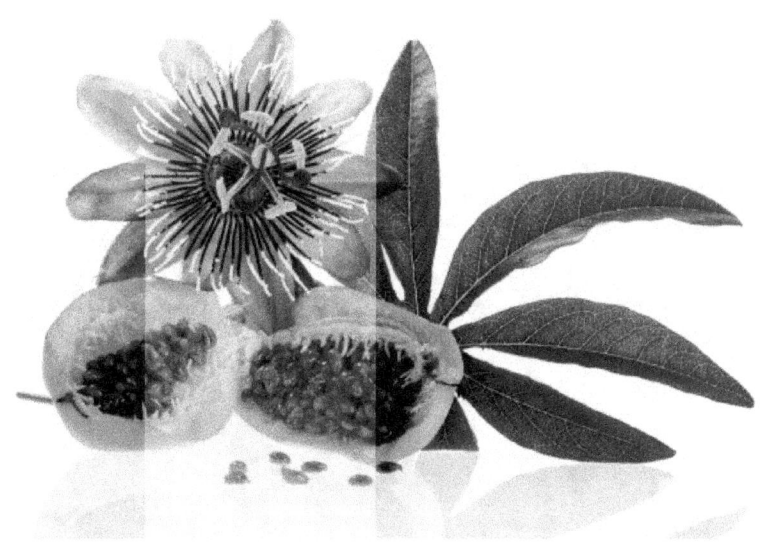

# IS PASSION FRUIT AND PASSION FLOWER THE SAME?

Yep – that's right!

The two most common fruiting passion flower are Passiflora edulis (which has both a purple and yellow species, along with hybrids) and Passiflora incarnata – also known as "Maypops". ... Passion fruit is sweet, tart, tangy, and downright delicious.

# VINE FOR WINE

Passionflower is a perennial vine that grows fairly quickly and is drought-tolerant.

The traditional systems of medicine in many countries mention about Passiflora for its use in breaking down alcohol addiction habits. Abrupt cessation of chronic administration of alcohol in human being and animals causes hyper-anxiety which is also manifested in the form of increased locomotor activity.

Dhawan K et al (2002) observed that in both, chronic and acute administrations, the benzoflavone moiety prevented significantly the expression of withdrawal effects of alcohol as there was a significant decrease in anxiety oriented behavior in mice that received benzoflavone moiety of P. incarnata.

The chronic administration of P. incarnata with alcohol had better preventive effects than the single acute treatment with P. incarnata in alcohol-dependent mice.

The benzoflavone moiety (BZF) reported from P. incarnata is the strongest aromatase enzyme inhibitor.

Inhibition of aromatase (a member of cytochrome P-450 enzyme family) prevents the metabolic conversion of testosterone to its metabolites, thereby, increasing the testosterone levels in the gonadal tissue, thus, increasing the free testosterone and decreasing free estrogen.

The BZF moiety isolated from aerial parts of P. incarnata acts:

(a) through its anti-aromatase function, and

(b) by eliminating estrogen's negative feedback loop.

The concomitant administration of BZF with alcohol maintains a high level of testosterone in the blood by stopping the aromatization of testosterone to estrogen.

Secondly, BZF also facilitates the body to produce more testosterone by eliminating the so-called 'negative feedback' loop, that otherwise reduces natural testosterone production due to alcoholism.

High testosterone accounts for normalization of behavioral changes, that otherwise appear, after cessation of chronic alcohol administration.

Thus, from these studies authors feel encouraged as the novel BZF moiety, being a highly potent antioxidant, and the strongest reported aromatase inhibitor, affords significant prevention against the hyper-anxiety induced by cessation of chronic administration of substances like alcohol.

The bioactive BZF prevents development of dependence of alcohol when administered concurrently with this, and upon cessation of alcohol, the BZF moiety maintains the high testosterone levels and prevents the occurrence of anxiety-manifested-withdrawal effects.

Even, an acute administration of BZF is able to block significantly the expression of withdrawal effects in mice rendered dependent upon ethanol, but at a significantly higher dose, i.e. 50 mg/kg, po.

Additionally, benzoflavone compounds can have strong anti-cancer effects as these are potent antioxidants, and can provide additional benefits of preventing hepatic cancers and liver cirrhosis, perhaps, the most alarming drawback of alcohol intake.

Dhawan K, Kumar S, Sharma A. Suppression of alcohol-cessation-oriented hyper-anxiety by the benzoflavone moiety of Passiflora incarnata Linneaus in mice. J Ethnopharmacol. 2002

Jul;81(2):239-44. doi: 10.1016/s0378-8741(02)00086-7. PMID: 12065157.

# PASSION TO TERMINATE CRIMES OF PASSION

Did you know that passionflower was once used by African American slave midwives to terminate pregnancies?

**Passionflower** should not be taken by **pregnant** women.

That's because it may stimulate the uterus and potentially induce labor.

While passionflower itself does not contain abortifacient properties, it seems that its use was primarily for its antispasmodic and sedative effects "for easing the fear, tension, anxiety, and pain of terminating a pregnancy

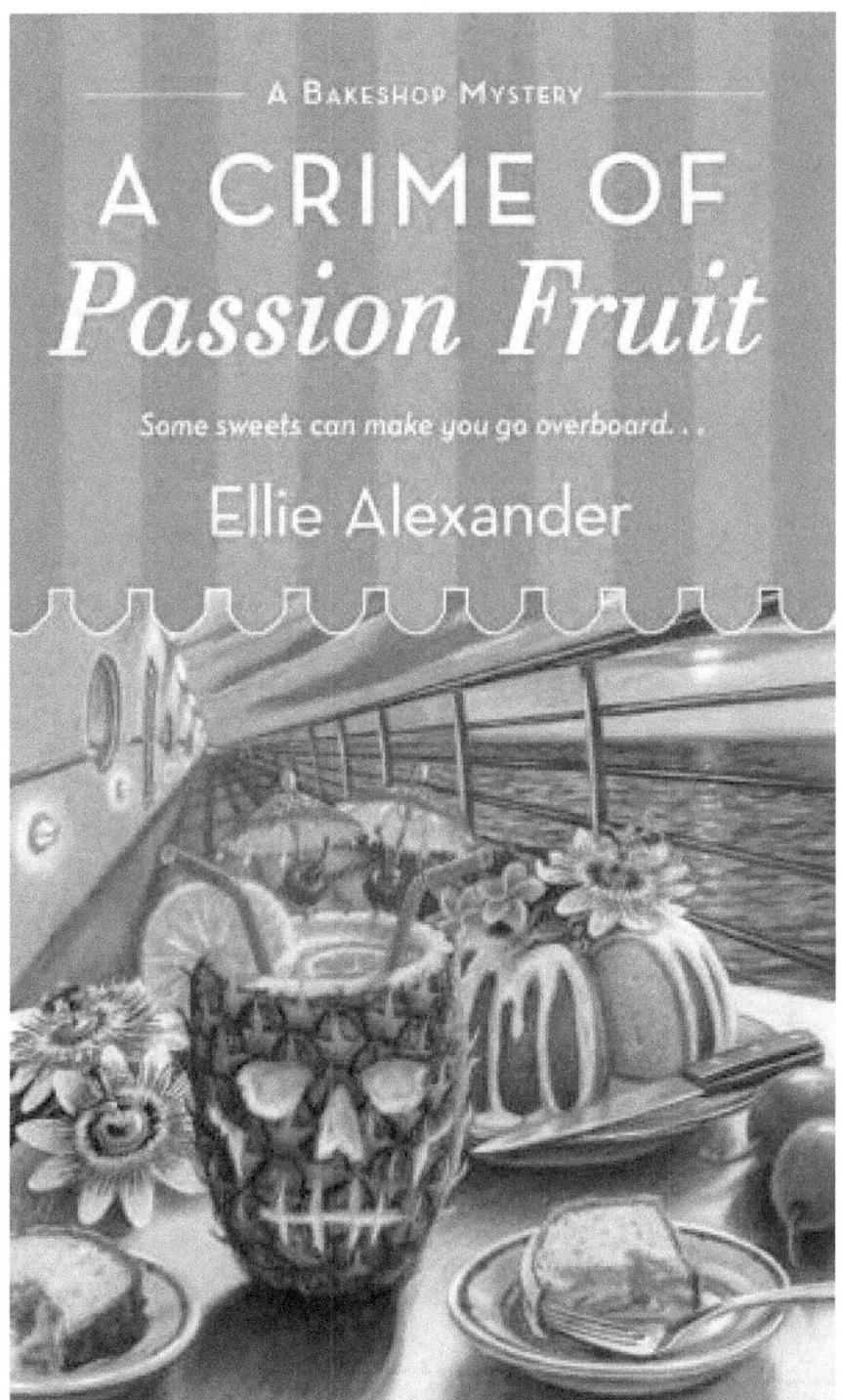

Figure 35. A Crime of Passion Fruit. (Bakeshop Murder Mystery #6) by Ellie Alexander. 2017

# ARE PASSION FRUITS AND PASSION FLOWERS THE SAME?

Basically, yes.

Passion fruit result from fertilised passion flowers but not all are used as fruit.

There are over 500 species of passion flowers (species name is Passiflora) but only about six are used for their fruit.

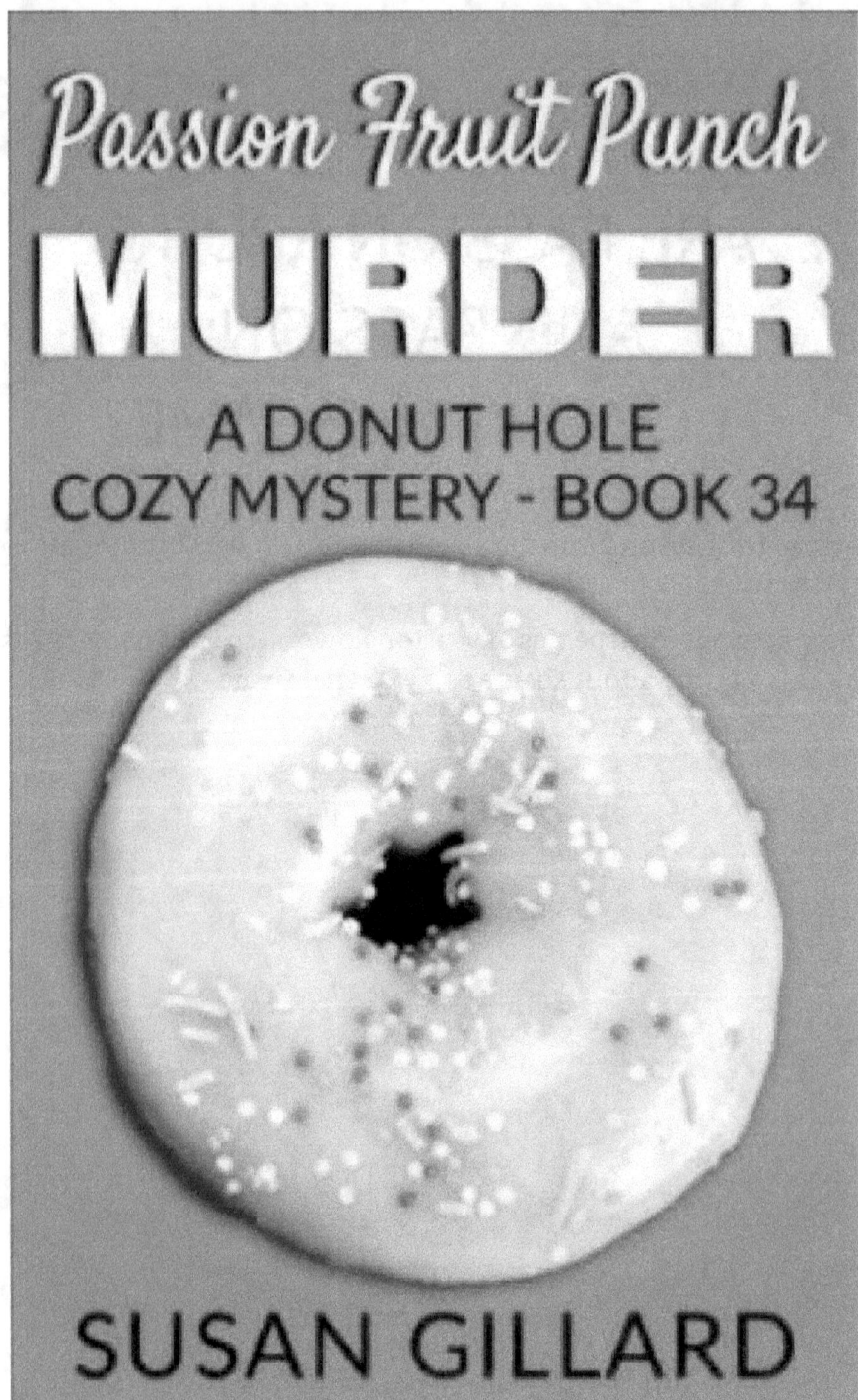

Figure 36. Passion Fruit Punch Murder by Susan Gillard (2017) (Donut Hole Cozy Mystery, book 34)

# IS TOO MUCH PASSION FRUIT BAD FOR YOU?

Purple passion fruit skin may also contain chemicals called cyanogenic glycosides. These can combine with enzymes to form the poison cyanide and are potentially poisonous in large amounts.

However, the fruit's hard outer skin isn't usually eaten and generally considered inedible.

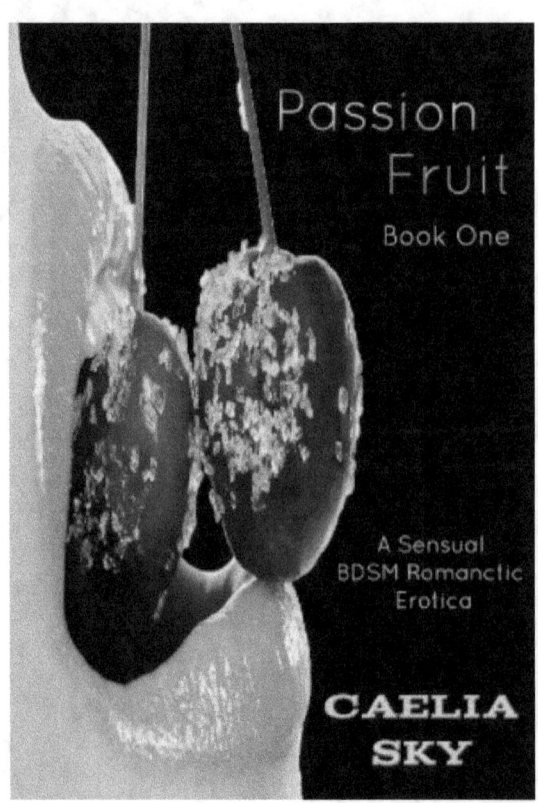

Figure 37. Passion Fruit (A Sensual Romantic) Sky Caelia.2017

# WHY DOES PASSION FRUIT MAKE YOU SLEEPY?

Some, though, contain high levels of caffeine, which will make it harder for you to fall asleep.

However, in passion fruit tea you can find Harman alkaloids- chemicals that relax your nervous system and make you tired, resulting in a more relaxed sleep.

# NIGHT, INSOMNIA STARTS TO SET

Epidemiological studies have estimated that about one third of the general population worldwide suffers from varying degrees of insomnia (Ohayon, 2002).

# U KNOW THAT U MUST GO TO BED

# AND YOU TRY TO TAKE SOME REST

The use of herbal medicines as an alternative treatment for insomnia symptoms has been increasing, because herbal products are readily accessible over the counter and are generally perceived to be safe (Gyllenhaal et al., 2000).

Gyllenhaal C, Merritt S, Peterson S, Block K, Gochenour T. 2000. Efficacy and safety of herbal stimulants and sedatives in sleep disorders. Sleep Med Rev 4: 229–251.

DR VIVEKANSHU VERMA FIST

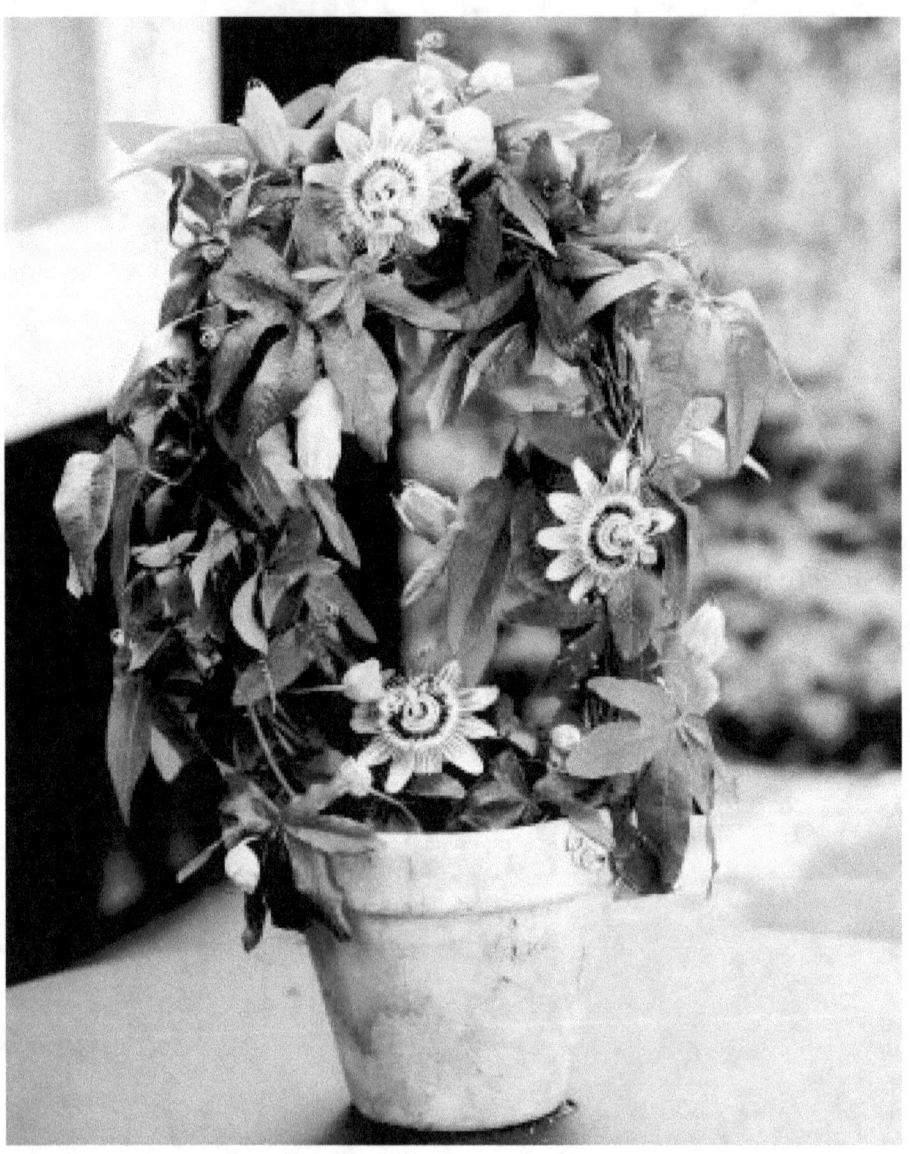

# SO EVERY NIGHT, ALONE IN BED

YOU SHED YOUR SILENT TEARS

CONSUMING ME, AS YOU SAID

However, many traditional sedative herbs, such as Passiflora incarnata, are employed to aid sleep without scientific support for their efficacy and safety for human consumption (Meoli et al., 2005).

Meoli AL, Rosen CR, Kristo D, Kohman M, Gooneratne N, Aguillard RE. 2005. Oral nonprescription treatment for insomnia: An evaluation of products with limited evidence. J Clin Sleep Med 1: 173–186.

DR VIVEKANSHU VERMA FIST

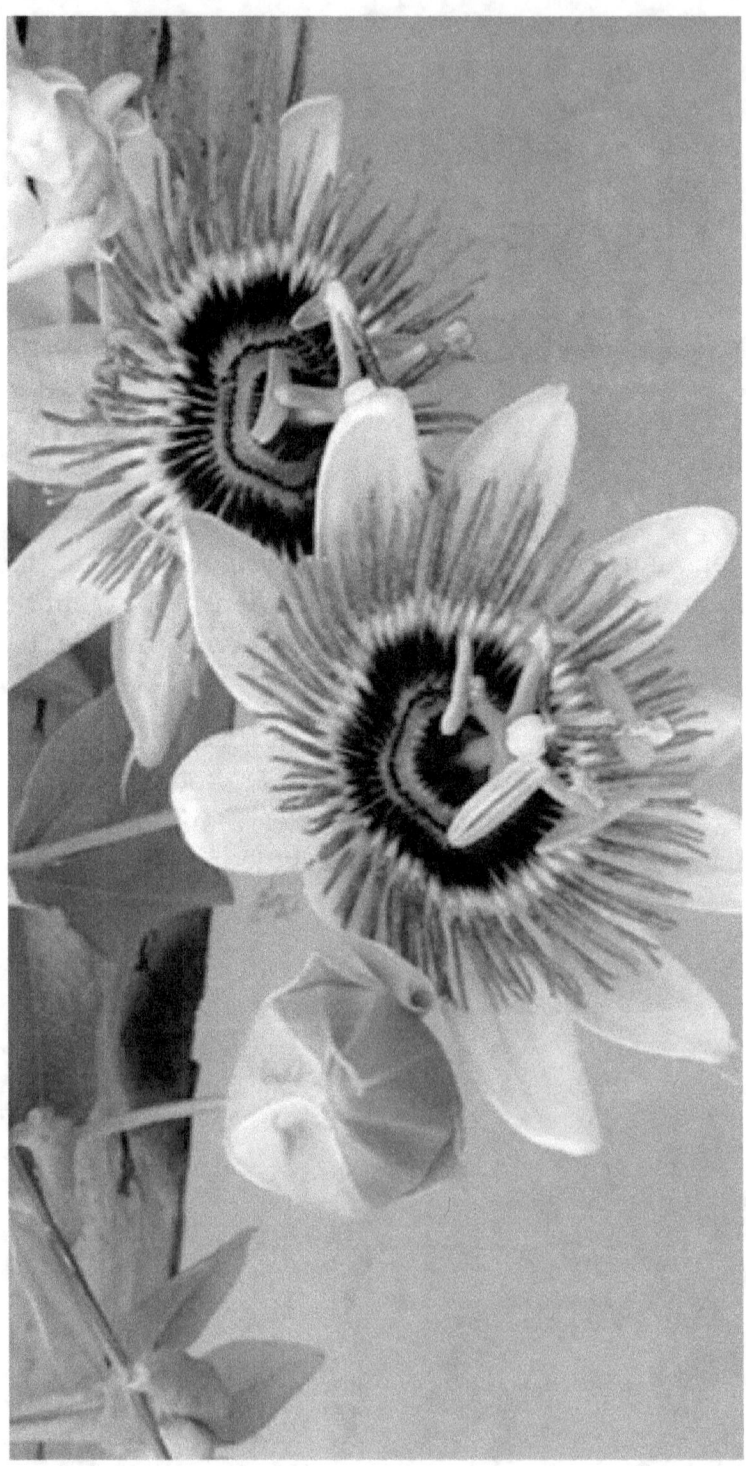

# DHAWAN'S PASSION

Passionflower is a folk anxiolytic and sedative used for the treatment of anxiety and insomnia symptoms, and has a history of use as a sedative in Brazil, Iraq, Turkey and North America as reported by Dhawan, et al. in serial case series from year 2001 to 2004, suggestive of Dhawan's passion for the passionflower (2001a,1b, 1c, 2003 2004).


Dhawan K, Kumar S, Sharma A. 2001b. Anxiolytic activity of aerial and underground parts of Passiflora incarnata. Fitoterapia 72: 922–926.

Dhawan K, Kumar S, Sharma A. 2001c. Comparative biological activity study on Passiflora incarnata and P. edulis. Fitoterapia 72: 698–702.

Dhawan K, Kumar S, Sharma A. 2003. Evaluation of central nervous system effects of Passiflora incarnata in experimental animals. Pharm Biol 41: 87–91.

To date, there is little scientifically validated evidence regarding either the constituents of Passiflora incarnate that are responsible for the speculated sedative and anxiolytic effects, or the plant's mechanism of action on sleep (Dhawan et al., 2004)

Dhawan K, Dhawan S, Sharma A. 2004. Passiflora: A review update. J Ethnopharmacol 94: 1–23. Dhawan K, Kumar S, Sharma A. 2001a. Anti-anxiety studies on extracts of Passiflora incarnata Linneaus. J Ethnopharmacol 78: 165–170.

# TEA OF PASSION

Ngan A et al (2011) in double-blind, placebo-controlled study of six sleep-diary measures analysed, sleep quality showed a significantly better rating for passionflower compared with placebo.

These findings suggest that the consumption of a low dose of Passiflora incarnata, in the form of tea, yields short-term subjective sleep benefits for healthy adults with mild fluctuations in sleep quality.

Citation: Ngan A, Conduit R. A double-blind, placebo-controlled investigation of the effects of Passiflora incarnata (passionflower) herbal tea on subjective sleep quality. Phytother Res. 2011 Aug;25(8):1153-9. doi: 10.1002/ptr.3400. Epub 2011 Feb 3. PMID: 21294203.

# GET HARM IN, PASS I, ON WINE

Harm All = harmol

Harm an = harmane

Harm aline = harmaline

Kenner D et al (1996) have ascribed the sedative effects of P. incarnata to indole alkaloids such as harmane and its relatives harmaline and harmol.

Kenner D, Requena Y. Botanical Medicine: A European Professional Perspective. Brookline MA: Paradigm Publications, 1996.

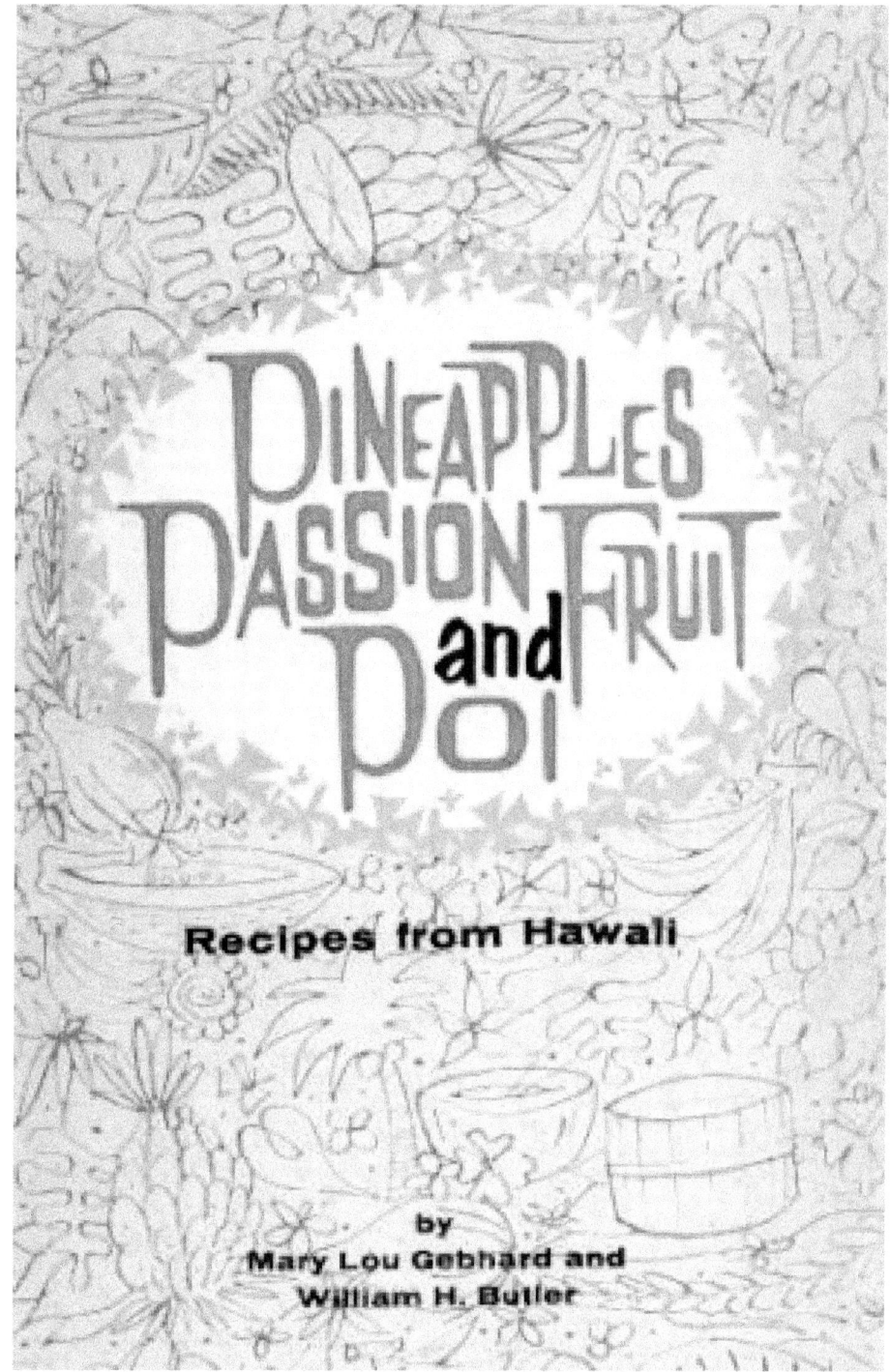

Figure 38. Pineapples, passion fruit and poi: recipes from Hawaii. Mary Lou Gebhard, William H. Butier.Year:1967

# DOES PASSION FRUIT MAKE YOU LOSE WEIGHT?

Passion fruit is a low-calorie, high-fiber fruit that may benefit blood pressure and insulin sensitivity, potentially making it ideal for weight loss.

# MENOPAUSE

Passion flower can help with symptoms like hot flashes and night sweats, but it's especially beneficial for mood-related symptoms like anxiety, depression, and emotional mood swings.

This is likely due to its calming effect on your nervous system and ability to increase GABA levels.

Elsas, S-M et al. "Passiflora incarnata L. (Passionflower) extracts elicit GABA currents in hippocampal neurons in vitro, and show anxiogenic and anticonvulsant effects in vivo, varying with extraction method." *Phytomedicine: international journal of phytotherapy and phytopharmacology* vol. 17,12 (2010): 940-9. doi:10.1016/j.phymed.2010.03.002

# HERB TO CURB PREOPERATIVE ANXIETY

Role of the flavonoid chrysin and even the pyrone derivative maltol to be responsible for the CNS effects of the plant.

Citation: Wolfman C, Viola H, Paladini A, Dajas F, Medina JH. Possible anxiolytic effects of chrysin, a central benzodiazepine receptor ligand isolated from Passiflora caerulea. Pharmacol Biochem Behav 1994;47:1–4.

Dental anxiety

Passion flower extract is extremely effective in relieving dental anxiety in patients.

Herbal drugs with sedative effects, such as Passion flower, have been used throughout the history as the anti-anxiety and sedative drugs.

In randomized- one sided blind clinical trial by Kaviani et al (2013), Passion flower was used as a sedative for dental anxiety, as an oral premedication, passiflora found significantly effective in reducing the anxiety. The latter is confirmed by statistical analysis which had the following results: The mean anxiety score prior and following drug intake was significantly different in the group receiving Passion flower extract.

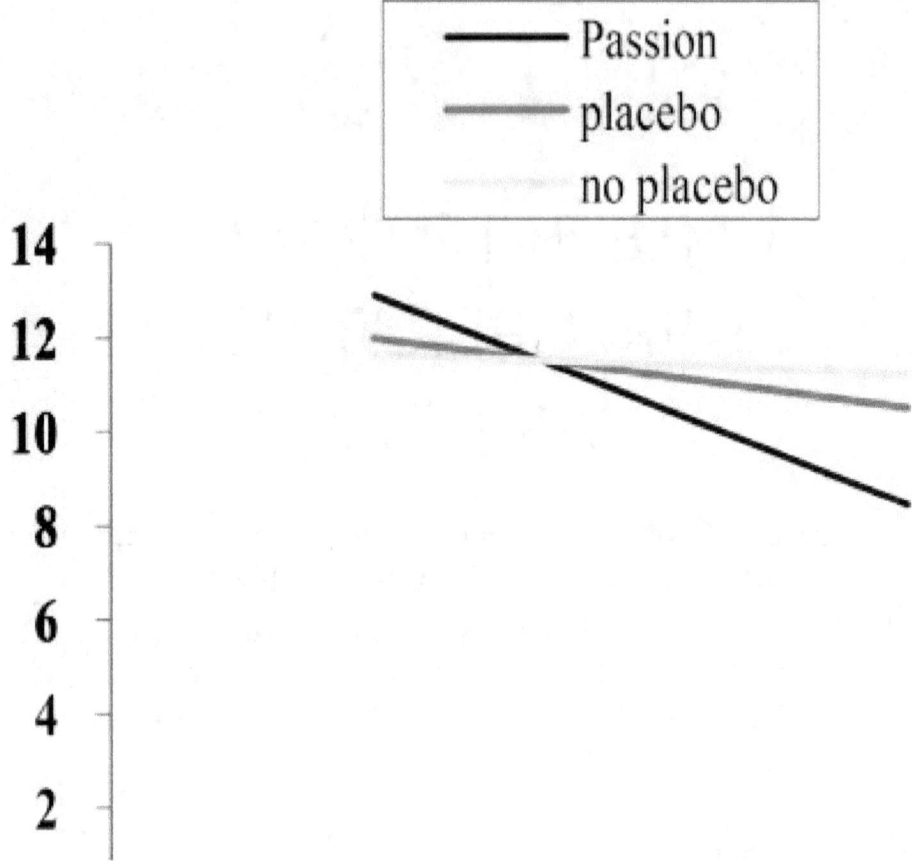

Figure 39. Efficacy of Passiflora in Reducing Dental Anxiety. Source: J Dent Med Univ Scien. 2013;14(2):68–72

Citation: Kaviani N, Tavakoli M, Tabanmehr MR, et al. The efficacy of Passiflora incarnata Linnaeus in Reducing Dental Anxiety in Patients undergoing periodontal treatment. J Dent Med Univ Scien. 2013;14(2):68–72

Sedative
Recently, the sedative and anxiolytic activities in Passiflora incarnata have been attributed to the benzodiazepine and γ-aminobutyric acid receptors-mediated biochemical processes in the body.

Citation: Loli F, Sato CM, Romanini CV, Viaggi Billas-Boas LD,

Moraes Santos CA, de Oliveira RMW. Possible involvement of GABAA-benzodiazepine receptor in the anxiolytic-like effect induced by Passiflora actinia extracts in mice. J Ethnopharmacol 2007;111:308–14.

Preoperative oral Passiflora incarnata reduces anxiety in ambulatory surgery patients

Many patients have preoperative anxiety; therefore, it would be desirable to develop a drug (preferably given orally) for premedication that is a strong anxiolytic with minimal psychomotor impairment. Benzodiazepines are presently the most commonly used class of anxiolytics.

Midazolam, because of its short duration of action, is the most popular; however, the oral formulation of midazolam is not approved in certain countries.

Herbal remedies are an increasingly popular form of therapy.

Citation: Krenn L. Passion Flower (Passiflora incarnata L.) – a reliable herbal sedative. Wien. Med. Wochenschr. 152, 404–406 (2002)

In outpatient surgery, administration of oral Passiflora incarnata as a premedication reduces anxiety without inducing sedation.

The current study Movafegh A et al (2008) demonstrated that patients who received oral premedication with Passiflora incarnata 500 mg (Passipy, IranDarouk) had a significant decrease in anxiety levels compared with patients who received placebo.

Movafegh A, Alizadeh R, Hajimohamadi F, Esfehani F, Nejatfar

M. Preoperative oral Passiflora incarnata reduces anxiety in ambulatory surgery patients: a double-blind, placebo-controlled study. Anesth Analg. 2008 Jun;106(6):1728-32. doi: 10.1213/ane.0b013e318172c3f9. PMID: 18499602.

# ANTICONVULSANT: PASSION SEIZES TO FIT

Passion flower (Passiflora incarnata) is used in traditional medicine of Europe and South America to treat seizure.

In study by Nassiri-Asl M et al (2007), anticonvulsant effects of hydro-alcoholic extract of Passiflora, Pasipay, were examined on mice. Pasipay at the dose of 0.4 mg/kg prolonged the onset time of seizure and decreased the duration of seizures. It seems that Pasipay could be useful for treatment absence seizure and these effects may be related to effect of it on GABAergic and opioid systems. More studies are needed in order to investigate its exact mechanism.

Nassiri-Asl M, Shariati-Rad S, Zamansoltani F. Anticonvulsant effects of aerial parts of Passiflora incarnata extract in mice: involvement of benzodiazepine and opioid receptors. BMC Complement Altern Med. 2007 Aug 8;7:26.

# ATTENTION TO PASSION

Passiflora may be a novel therapeutic agent for the treatment of ADHD (Attention-deficit hyperactivity disorder).

first double-blind, controlled trial of passiflora in the treatment of ADHD done by Akhundzadeh S et al (2005) observed that tablets of passiflora and methylphenidate are effective in the treatment of ADHD. No significant difference was observed between the two protocols at the end of the trial. Nevertheless, in the passiflora group, but not the methylphenidate group, significant effects were observed by week 2 and indicates a rapid onset of action for Passiflora. In addition, the substantially lower incidence of decreased appetite and anxiety/nervousness could be an important advantage of Passiflora.

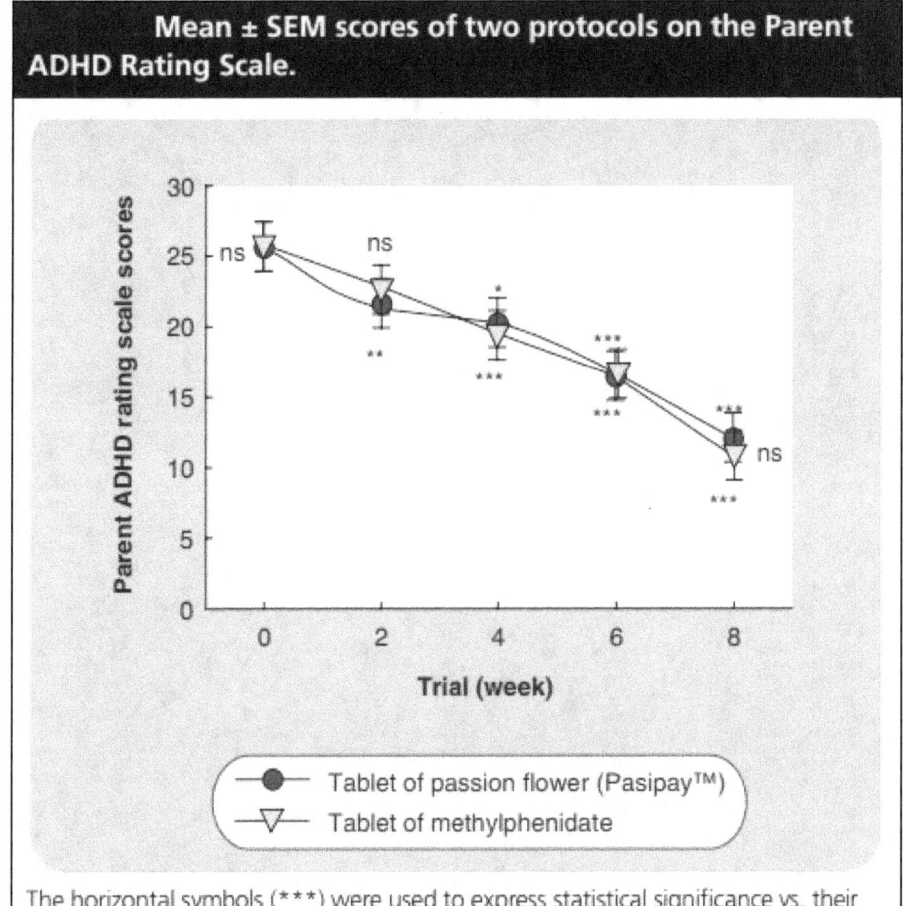

Figure 40. Passiflora incarnata in treatment of attention-deficit hyperactivity disorder in children and adolescents. Source: Akhundzadeh S, Mohammadi MR, Momeni F. Therapy. 2005;2:609–614.

The limitations of the above study, including the lack of a placebo group, using only a fixed dose of passiflora, the small number of participants and the short period of follow-up should be considered; therefore, further research in this area is needed.

Akhundzadeh S, Mohammadi MR, Momeni F. Passiflora incarnata in treatment of attention-deficit hyperactivity disorder in children and adolescents. Therapy. 2005;2:609–614.

# HYPERTENSION, DOWN BY PASSION

Extracts of the family Passifloraceae are known to have several important physiological effects on mammals.

Ichimura T et al (2006) observed that orally administered methanol extract of *Passiflora edulis* significantly lowered systolic blood pressure in Rats.

Passiflora edulis rind, which remains as an unused resource after squeezing juice from the fruits, was studied as antihypertensive agent.

It has been proposed that GABA, one of the depressive neurotransmitters in the central nervous system, play an important physiological role in the regulation of cardiovascular function.

Since 50 mg of Passiflora edulis rind extract contains 0.22 mg of GABA, estimated from the data with the amino acid analyzer, we consider that the extract contains a high enough concentration of GABA to decrease blood pressure.

Luteolin-6-Cchinovoside and luteolin-6-C-fucoside have been isolated from leaves of Passiflora edulis. Passiflora Flavonoids exhibit diverse biological effects, including inhibition of protein kinase C, inhibition of cyclic nucleotide phosphodiesterase, decrease in $Ca^{2+}$ uptake, and vasodilatory actions.

Citation: Ichimura T, Yamanaka A, Ichiba T, Toyokawa T, Kamada Y, Tamamura T, Maruyama S. Antihypertensive effect of an extract of Passiflora edulis rind in spontaneously hypertensive rats. Biosci Biotechnol Biochem. 2006;70:718-721. doi:10.1271/bbb.70.718

www.ingramcontent.com/pod-product-compliance
Lightning Source LLC
Chambersburg PA
CBHW060844220526
45466CB00003B/1241